Crystals for Beginners

Why Crystals and Gemstones Have a Magical Healing Power and How to Make Them Work to Get Health and Positive Energy in Your Life

a licensed professional before attempting any techniques outlined in this book.

By reading this document, the reader agrees that under no circumstances is the author responsible for any losses, direct or indirect, which are incurred as a result of the use of information contained within this document, including, but not limited to, — errors, omissions, or inaccuracies.

Table of Contents

Introduction

Whether to adorn the crowns of powerful kings and queens, to give power to a mage's staff, or to channel energy when building and casting spells, crystals have always been associated with magic, power, and mysterious mystic forces. Although not as exaggerated as in fantasy books and games, crystals do carry power with them, as well as deep symbolism that goes back to the dawn of time. There is a whole world to discover when it comes to crystals, and it can be daunting and a little scary to explore, especially if you don't know where to start. That is precisely what this book is for. Whether you're a fresh new explorer carefully testing the waters for the first time or an experienced spelunker who's been diving in and out of the hidden nooks and crannies of the crystal world for years, this book will help you understand crystals a bit better.

Not only will this book give an explanation on how crystals work, where they come from, what they look like, and what they do, but it will also show you how you can use crystals to improve your own life from aligning chakras and boosting the effects of meditation to using crystals in simple ways to alleviate stress and depression and improving almost all aspects of your everyday life.

To take it a step further, this book will help guide you in building your own personal crystal collection and one that works best for you, and it will teach you how to care for and maintain your collection, as well as how to best use it to its full potential.

Furthermore, you will be reading a list of the most prominent and important crystals with clear descriptions, where they come from, and how they can be used, making it easy to identify your crystals.

Chapter 1: What Are Crystals?

Before you can properly understand how crystals work and what they can do for you, it's important to understand what they are and where they come from. The minerals and formation processes can have an influence on the appearance and the abilities of crystals.

A Brief History of Crystals

Crystals have been a part of life since the dawn of our species, and records of the use of crystals can be dated all the way back to the ancient Sumerians. The Sumerians used crystals in almost all of their magic formulas. Bracelets with amber beads have been found in Britain that date back 10,000 years. Amber is not naturally found in England, meaning they have traveled long distances to get there. This shows us that amber was important enough to the people that they would carry these beads all the way with them. The ancient Egyptians often used stones such as lapis lazuli, emerald, and clear quartz for their jewelry and commonly carved grave masks out of these gemstones.

The use of crystals and gemstones became especially popular in ancient Greece, and most of the crystal names we use today originate from this era. Even the word crystal comes from the Greek word *krustallos* meaning "ice". They used this word because the people believed that crystals were ice frozen so solidly that they would never melt. Different crystals were often associated with the gods and used in religious rituals and to decorate their temples. The Greeks also had many superstitions that involved crystals, such as wearing amethyst to avoid getting drunk or having a hangover or rubbing hematite (a crystal associated with Ares, the god of war) all over their bodies before battle believing it would make them invulnerable from then on.

Most religious texts such as the Koran and the Bible refer to crystals and gemstones several times, and many religious rituals incorporate crystals or assign a significant meaning to certain types of crystals. In many cultures, green stones were a symbol of life, and people were often buried with one of these stones over their heart.

The Chinese culture has always put special emphasis on jade, recognizing it as a kidney healing stone, and around 1,000 years ago, emperors were often buried in jade armor. Instruments in the form of chimes were commonly made and hung in homes and places of business, and even some of the characters in Chinese writing were designed to resemble jade beads.

Crystals no longer have such a deep cultural and significance as they used to, though they are still a powerful tool when it comes to healing and improving the lives of those who use them. Some of the symbolism connected with stones is still incorporated into modern culture in small ways, especially in books and films, such as a green stone being a core element of restoring life to a dying world or returning a broken-off shard to a magical crystal that keeps the world in balance. Crystals are also still a popular subject for scientists to study, and there are many scholarly courses and professional careers that concern the use of crystals and their abilities.

What Is a Crystal?

The term *crystal* or *crystalline* generally refers to a solid material in which clusters of atoms are arranged together in a regular geometric pattern, often resulting in prominent facets (though not always). By piling these clusters of atoms together in a repeating pattern, the crystal will grow larger. This pattern extends outward in three dimensions. Most crystals are rock formations, but there are some exceptions such as ice crystals and sugar. The type of pattern and structure of the atom cluster sets the type of crystal and is usually affected by how the crystal forms. The most common type of crystal found in everyday life is salt, and it can easily be used in experiments in growing crystals.

Gemstones

The term *gemstone* often comes to mind when talking about crystals, but there is a difference between a gemstone and a crystal. Gemstones are rare rock formations that can be used for decoration and jewelry and classified as *precious* or *semi-precious*, while crystals are structures of atoms arranged in a geometric pattern that extend into three dimensions. Most gemstones, such as diamonds, amber, and sapphire, are considered forms of crystal, but not all types of crystals are considered gemstones. Just as with crystals, gemstones can have a base construction of minerals or a more organic origin, as can be seen with amber. It can be especially important to know the difference between the two when buying crystals, as you might not be buying what you expect, and gemstones are usually more expensive than crystals.

How Do Crystals Form?

There are several ways by which crystals form. The general process is called *crystallization*. The most common form of crystallization is growing it from a liquid. As a liquid filled with minerals and other matter molecules condenses into gas form, the mineral molecules will remain solid and start packing themselves together in an attempt to remain stable, and a crystal is formed. The more the water condenses, the more molecules that will be packed together and the larger the crystal becomes. Not all molecules will form crystals, and the type of minerals present in the liquid will determine the color, density, shape, and type of crystal. If a solid structure is already present (i.e. a rock standing in a pool of mineral-rich water), the molecules will cling to it and the crystal formation will grow into this structure.

Another way crystals are formed is by cooling liquids. In much the same way, different types of molecules cluster together in a repeating pattern to form the crystals. The most common occurrence is molten lava cooling down, forming crystals within the rocks, which is one of the reasons why crystals are often abundant in areas with many volcanoes and tectonic plates nearby.

In some rare occasions, crystals can be formed by compressing gas into a solid form. This requires incredibly large amounts of pressure and usually takes hundreds of years to form a decently-sized crystal. Diamonds are formed by compressing carbon in this way, and it is because of the rarity of the right conditions and the amount of time it takes to form a diamond that makes them so incredibly expensive.

Outside factors such as general temperature, available space, available minerals, cooling speed, and humidity, as well as many other minor factors, will help determine the type of crystal that will form.

Where Do Crystals Come From?

Different crystals can be found in various regions due to the specific minerals and other elements available, but there are certain types of places where crystals tend to grow. Crystals generally form in rocky areas and under the ground, especially if these places remain undisturbed. Most of the earth's bedrock is one form of a crystal or another. As mentioned above, some crystals are formed within cooling lava, and this is where most of the world's crystals and gemstones are found. Lava comes from beneath the earth's crust and is sometimes pushed through to the surface, forming layers. The movement of the earth's tectonic plates have a similar effect, and this is how new crystals are created. Some crystals are formed immediately as the lava on the surface cools quickly, but others take much longer to form further down where the lava cools at a much slower pace. The speed at which a crystal is formed usually determines its size.

In some cases, the movement of the lava or earth creates empty spaces where water vapors are condensed into a mineral-rich liquid which will eventually grow into different crystals. Many underground caverns are damp and desolate enough that large clusters of crystals can grow for hundreds of years. Geodes form when gas or liquid is allowed to crystallize in a small cavity inside rocks and stones. Agate is a very common crystal to find inside geodes, and the majority of the world's geodes will have at least one or two layers of agate as a crust. In some cases, the cavity inside a geode will be completely filled with crystallized chalcedony and you will have a solid piece of agate, but it is also possible that you will have several layers of agate and another type of crystal, usually quartz, growing in the very center of the geode.

In some areas that have mineral-rich earth, it is possible to find small crystals scattered about or in the uppermost layer of the ground. The area will determine the types of crystals that can be found. Individual crystals are more likely than clusters, and many of these crystals will go unnoticed in their raw form. In some sandy areas, it is possible to find crystal formations such as desert roses and sand crystals. There are also a few places in the world where the sand consists of tiny crystals that are worn down. Quartz is an important mineral in sand formation, and it is often found that many sand grains are, in fact, quartz crystals.

There are also a few types of crystals that are grown from organic matter, such as amber, which is crystallized tree sap, or calcite and aragonite, which are produced by most mollusks.

Crystal Lattice

The term *crystal lattice* refers to the specific type of three-dimensional pattern in which the atoms are connected to form the crystal, and it can also be called the structure of the crystal. The lattice of a crystal is a key component in classifying crystals, as each type of crystal has a unique lattice. Many outside influences such as radiation, exposure to the elements, the way in which the crystal forms, and chemical impurities can affect the shape, color, and size of a crystal, but the lattice will remain the same. This is why two stones that look completely different from each other in color and shape can still be classified as the same type of crystal. The lattice will determine the number of faces (flat surfaces that form the shape of the crystal) a crystal has, as well as how they are placed in relation to each other.

As mentioned above, all crystals are formed through repeating geometric patterns, and there are seven specific types of patterns that occur. These types are lattice types. Crystal structures can be reduced to the smallest possible form of the pattern that can be repeated in three dimensions. This singular part of the lattice is called the *unit cell*, and it forms the base of the lattice used to create a crystal. A unit cell consists of a few atoms packed together in a set geometric shape which is repeated over and over again to form the lattice of the crystal. The three dimensions in which the pattern is repeated roughly indicate the different directions that the growth of the crystal takes place. The growth in the three dimensions is often represented by *crystallographic axes*, imaginary lines that intersect at 90-degree angles in the center of the crystal lattice. There are three axes used to represent the dimensions; they are simply referred to as the x-axis, y-axis, and z-axis, and they are usually perfectly perpendicular to each other. This set of axes is used frequently in science and math, but it also forms the core of 3D editing programs. In such programs, an object can be moved or altered forward and backward, to the left and right, and up and down, and each of these types of direction is indicated by an axis. The same concept is applied to a crystal lattice. The symmetry along each axis plays a large role in determining the type of lattice in a crystal.

Symmetry is an important element of crystal lattices. It refers to how the pattern is repeated, specifically how one cell unit is connected to the next. There are two different types of symmetry: translational symmetry and point symmetry. Translational symmetry is where the pattern is repeated simply through movement along a line or within a certain volume. As an example, if a cube-shaped cell unit is repeated by placing the units next to or on top of each other, translational symmetry is used to form a cubic lattice. Point symmetry is where the repetition occurs around a central point, such as in the cases of rotation, reflection, and inversion, along with others. An example of point symmetry is when a triangular unit cell is rotated around a central point in all three dimensions to form a triangle-based pyramid.

The initial shape of the cell unit and the type of symmetry determines the type of lattice that will be formed. Below we will go over the different types of crystal lattice in detail:

1. *Isometric*

This is also often called the cubic lattice, and it's built on a square-shaped cell unit. In this case, the crystallographic axes have perfect symmetry and are usually the same length. The axes can also often be applied diagonally and still be perfectly symmetrical. The different planes of the crystal that run parallel with each other will always be matched in shape and size. Cube- and diamond-shaped crystals are the most common results of this lattice type. Good examples of crystals with an isometric type lattice are magnetite and garnet.

2. *Hexagonal*

The hexagonal lattice system has a fourth axis. One axis runs vertically, but rather than two horizontal lines cutting each other to form four 90-degree corners, three lines meet each other to form three 120-degree corners. These three lines are no longer perpendicular to each other but are still perpendicular to the vertical line. The three 120-degree axes are usually symmetric and of equal length, while the fourth, perpendicular line can be longer or shorter. This lattice type results in crystals with eight faces, and crystals usually form prisms and pyramids with a six-sided base. The most common crystals with a hexagonal type lattice are high quartz, beryl, and apatite.

3. Tetragonal

Similar to the isometric system, this lattice system has three axes that meet in 90-degree corners. One of the axes, however, can be extended or shortened, forming a rectangular shape. Crystals with this type of lattice tend to have six faces, where the base and opposite face form a perfect square shape and the other four faces form rectangles. Some good examples of these types of crystals are cassiterite and zircon.

4. Rhombohedral

This system is similar to both the tetragonal system by having three perpendicular (meaning they all form 90-degree corners) axes, with one axis longer or shorter than the other two. It also has six faces, but rather than forming a perfectly square base, these crystals tend to form a base that is the shape of a diamond (also called a rhombus). Crystals with this type of lattice include low quartz, tourmaline, and dolomite.

5. Orthorhombic

This is another lattice system with three axes that meet perpendicularly, but unlike the other systems, none of the three axes are of the same length. These crystals tend to have six faces, but the base face forms an irregular four-sided shape that isn't a square, rectangle, or diamond. These crystals can also form tube and oblong spherical type shapes. Crystals commonly identified by this lattice system are barite and olivine.

6. Monoclinic

This system uses three axes as well, but while the vertical axis meets the other two at a 90-degree angle, the two vertical axes meet each other at a corner that can be either larger or smaller than 90 degrees. These types of crystals usually consist of six faces and form long prisms. This is a very common lattice system for crystals, and some of the best examples are azurite, malachite, and pyroxene.

7. Triclinical

In this system, none of the three axes meet each other at a 90-degree angle. Unlike the six other lattice types, there is no symmetry to these crystals, and there are no faces that will mirror each other. There is also no regulation to the number of faces these crystals will have, although they do tend to be tubular. Some examples of triclinical crystals are axinite and plagioclase.

Crystal Shapes

A big part of crystal identification is the shape. The crystal lattice determines the potential types of shapes which can be identified by the number of faces, faces that mirror each other, and the basic symmetry of the crystal.

Although most crystals don't form geometrically perfect shapes, and crystals of the same type will not be identical in shape and size, they will conform to the same basic shape type. There are eleven basic shape types in which crystals can be classified.

1. *Monohedron*

This shape is also a *pedion,* and it consists of an undetermined number of faces that are each geometrically unique. None of the faces are parallel or mirror each other in any way. This shape is the result of a triclinic lattice.

2. Parallelohedron

This shape is another result of a triclinical lattice and can also be referred to as a *pinacoid*. This shape has two faces that run parallel to one another and are geometrically the same 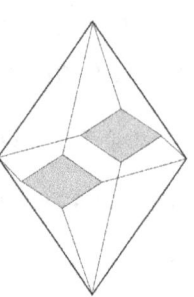 shape. These two faces might be a reflection or inversion of each other, but they are not perfectly mirrored.

3. *Dihedron*

A dihedron contains two faces that geometrically match and can either be related to each other through reflection or rotation. If these two faces are a simple reflection or rotation on 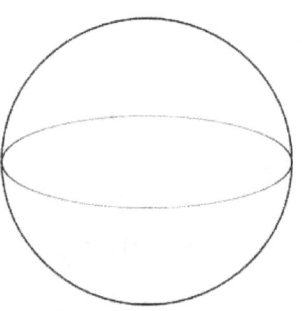 only one axis, the dihedron will form a roughly dome-shaped crystal. If the two faces run along more than one rotational axis, the dihedron will form a more sphere-shaped crystal. The dihedron shape is caused by a monoclinic lattice type.

4. *Disphenoid*

The disphenoid shape consists of two sets of faces that are geometrically the same in shape and size, but they do not run parallel with each other. 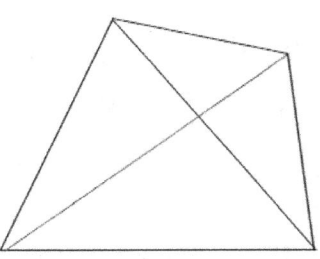 These shapes share symmetry through rotation and are connected by one of their edges. An orthorhombic lattice can result in a rhombic disphenoid, while a tetragonal lattice can result in a tetragonal disphenoid.

5. *Prism*

A prism consists completely of sets of mirroring faces that are both geometrically identical and run parallel to each other. The two faces of each mirroring set are on opposite sides of the crystal, and all the sets are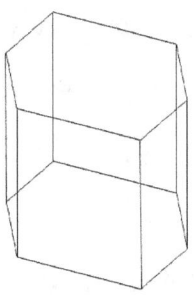

reflected around the same axis. Usually, one set will form the base, which can be almost any basic shape, such as a square, triangle, or hexagon, while the other sets will all be rectangular. These rectangular faces that meet the edges of the base face at 90-degree angles will form a tube-like shape for the crystal. Prisms are a result of a monoclinic lattice system.

6. *Pyramid*

The pyramid shape consists of a base face and a set of three, four, six, eight, or twelve faces that do not run parallel to each other but meet in a point instead. Usually, the crystal will have a base face that 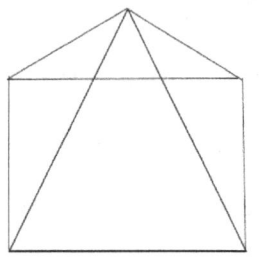 can have one of several shapes, such as a square or triangle, with triangular shapes along each edge that will meet each other at the apex of the crystal. The shape of the base face will determine the type of pyramid and the number of faces in the set, and it is determined by the lattice type. The hexagonal, tetragonal, and orthorhombic lattice types are capable of producing pyramid-shaped crystals.

7. *Dipyramid*

This shape basically consists of two pyramids connected base to base with an apex at both ends. The two pyramids share the same base in the middle of the crystal and are a reflection of each other. A dipyramid shape can have a 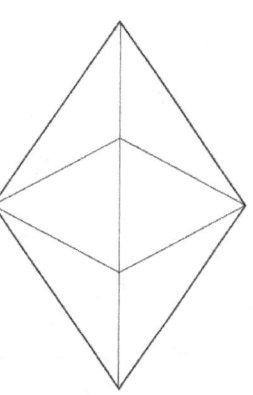 hexagonal, tetragonal, or orthorhombic lattice type, and the shape of the shared base will determine the type of dipyramid shape of the crystal. Each of the faces of a dipyramid will be triangular in shape as well, and a dipyramid will have twice as many faces as a pyramid with the same base.

8. *Trapezohedron*

A trapezohedron looks similar to a dipyramid but has significant differences. Firstly, a trapezohedron does not have a shared base between the two apexes of the shape. Rather than triangular shapes, each face will have a trapezoidal (four sides that are not perpendicular) shape. The type of trapezohedron will be determined by the amount of faces on each side (i.e. a

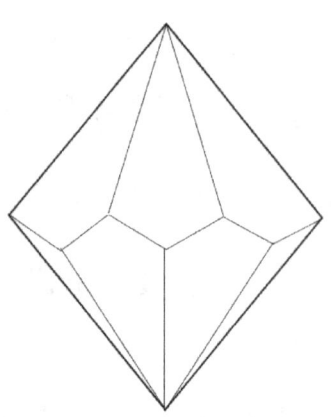

trigonal trapezoid will have six faces in total, with three at the top and three at the bottom). A tetragonal trapezohedron will have four faces on both sides for a total of eight faces, and a hexagonal trapezohedron will have six faces on both sides, resulting in 12 faces. This shape can have a tetragonal or hexagonal lattice.

9. *Scalenohedron*

Like a trapezohedron, the scalenohedron resembles two pyramids but will have no base shape in the middle of the crystal. Unlike the trapezohedron, however, each of the faces of the crystal will be in the shape of a

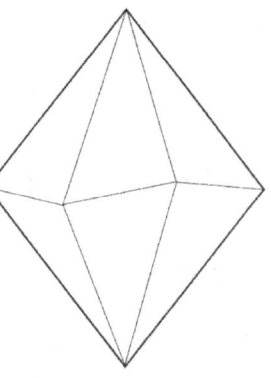

scalene triangle, meaning two of the corners of the triangle are smaller than 90 degrees and the other is larger than 90 degrees. A scalenohedron will have either eight or twelve faces that are grouped in symmetrical pairs. This shape can be the result of a hexagonal or tetragonal lattice.

10. *Rhombohedron*

This shape consists of six diamond-shaped faces and looks like a cube that is turned to stand upright on one corner and has been flattened or elongated along

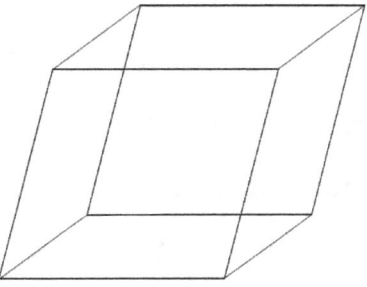

its diagonal axis. This shape can have a rhombohedral or hexagonal lattice type. An important trademark is that opposing sides of the rhombohedron are geometrically the same in shape and size and run parallel to each other; they are not a reflection of each other along a vertical or horizontal axis.

11. *Tetrahedron*

The tetrahedron is a shape composed of four triangular shapes. The lattice of the crystal will determine the type of tetrahedron and the shape of the triangle. A tetrahedron 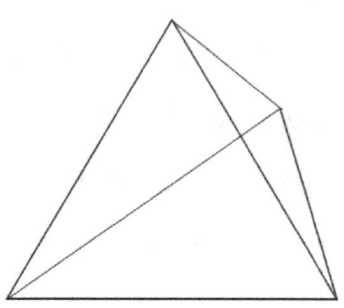 with an isometric lattice will consist of four equilateral (all three sides are the same length and all three corners are 60 degrees) triangles that are identical. A tetragonal lattice system will result in four identical triangles that each have two sides of the same length, also known as an isosceles triangle. A crystal with an orthorhombic lattice will have two sets of matching isosceles triangles.

Crystal Colors

Color is a large part of identifying crystals. The color of a crystal is mainly determined by the types of minerals the crystal is grown from, although many outside influences during the forming of a crystal can have a huge influence. Each crystal type has a certain lattice, growth process, and mineral composition, and each will have a specific color associated with it. Quartz is a good example in this case; a pure quartz crystal will be completely colorless, but outside influences can alter this. Amethyst is a member of the quartz family but gains its purple color from trace elements of iron within the crystal. Rose quartz is pink due to traces of titanium or manganese, and smoky quartz is brown because specific color centers are activated when traces of aluminum within the crystal are exposed to natural radiation transmitted by specific types of stone. Some crystal types will change colors if repeatedly exposed to light, such as realgar, which can change from red to yellow. Some crystals will change colors when viewed in different types of light, and crystals such as opal will reflect different colors when looked at from different angles. Many crystals and gemstones are often treated with intense heat when being transformed into jewelry as high temperatures can deepen the color of certain types.

These changes due to outside elements can be more intense in some crystal types and cause significant differences as seen with the quartz example, but in other crystal types, these changes are quite small, such as with azurite, where the exact hue of blue can be affected.

Certain colors will always be associated with specific elements and minerals, such as copper that will result in blue or green stones, iron that is usually associated with red and brown, and cobalt and manganese which can cause a pink hue. Due to this, certain colors in crystals will be linked to specific healing properties and uses.

Opacity and Transparency

When discussing the appearance of crystals, terms such as *opaque, translucent,* and *transparent* are bound to pop up. These three terms have everything to do with how much light passes through a crystal or how much light it reflects back. If a crystal is transparent, it means that all light passes through the crystal and you can see right through it with perfect clarity, just like glass. An opaque crystal reflects back all light and isn't see-through whatsoever. The term translucent is used when a crystal lets some light pass through but not all. These crystals can be partially seen through and are usually blurry.

The translucency of a crystal is mostly determined by the elements it is formed from but, once again, outside influences can have an effect on this. In some cases, it is even possible for one crystal to have varying degrees of translucency. Agate is a good example, as one ring can be completely transparent while the next can be only slightly translucent, bordering on opaque. Some crystal types have very reflective surfaces, though they do not fall into a classification of their own. Crystals with reflective surfaces can still be transparent, translucent, or opaque, depending on how much can be seen through the crystal beyond the reflection.

Stripes and Rings

Many crystal types such as tiger's eye, agate, and malachite are most easily recognized by their various layers of stripes and rings, and the intensity in the variations between the layers can often influence the value of these stones. All crystals, no matter how big or small, are formed in layers which are usually not noticeable by the human eye. Severe changes in the environment, such as temperature changes, the sudden appearance of new minerals, or a change in pressure, can cause small changes in the properties of a crystal, resulting in the current layer being a little bit different from the previous layer. Some minerals, such as chalcedony, are more sensitive to these changes and will form clearly varying layers more easily than others, becoming beautifully layered agate. The most common differences between layers are a change in the exact hue or intensity of the crystal's natural color or a shift in the opacity in each layer. Radical changes such as a blue and red layer in the same stone are not a natural occurrence. Many of these striped or ringed crystals are cut and polished in a way that will show off these layers as much as possible.

Imperfections

Growing crystals is a very complicated and precise process, and it's only natural for a few mistakes to be made here and there. Imperfections can have a large influence on the appearance and structural integrity of a crystal and make them either more or less valuable. Certain impurities can even have an influence on the healing properties of a crystal. There are different types of imperfections, namely impurities, interstitial defects, vacancy defects, displacement, and twinning. Impurities occur when an unwanted or incorrect type of atom is present within a crystal. A good example is lapis lazuli; this crystal is mostly made out of lazurite, but clusters of calcite and pyrite cause white and gold speckles. In the case of lapis lazuli, these impurities are preferred and make the crystal more valuable.

Interstitial defects happen when there is an extra atom within the lattice of the crystal where it doesn't belong.

In opaque crystals, this is simply noticed by a small part that is a bit harder than the rest. In transparent and translucent crystals, this defect is more easily noticeable. This defect can be seen as a small part of the crystal looking more dense and opaque than the rest of it. Depending on the frequency and placement of these extra atoms, it can create misty swirls or darker veins within the crystal. Impurities can also be a type of interstitial defect if a different type of atom is squeezed into a space where no atoms belong.

A vacancy defect is the complete opposite and happens when there is an atom missing in the lattice pattern. A large number of vacancies spread throughout the crystal can cause it to be softer and more fragile than usual, but this is very rare. In most cases, the vacancies are small, and the structure of the atoms surrounding the vacancy will assure that the crystal does not collapse in on itself.

Dislocation occurs when there is a sudden shift in the lattice pattern of a crystal. This usually means that there is a partial plain or row added or removed from the pattern, and the rest of the lattice then moves slightly to maintain the stability of the crystal. In some cases, this can cause faint bends and wobbles in normally flat and straight surfaces on the crystal. These are usually so small, however, that they can't be seen by the naked eye.

Twinning basically happens when crystals of the same type are clustered too closely together and grow into one crystal. These are individual crystals that share some points in their lattice. A good example is pyrite, which has a cube shape. In the case of twinned pyrite, you will be able to see each individual cube, but they will be intersecting. These squares can either simply share a face, in which case they will simply look like two cubes roughly glued together, or they can penetrate each other, causing corners and edges of one cube to disappear into or grow out of the faces of the other cubes.

Cutting and Polishing

Crystals aren't always sold in the same state they are found in; they often go through a cleaning, cutting, and polishing process. When crystals are found or mined, they are treated beforehand to enhance their appearance, especially if they are destined to become jewelry. There are many different methods to cut and polish gems, but almost all involve the use of other, harder gemstones and crystals. Special tools such as saw-blades, grinders, and sandpaper are reinforced or created using incredibly hard crystals like diamond to cut and polish crystals into different shapes. Certain shapes also have special meanings and powers when used for healing. There are certain types of cuts that are used on more precious gemstones to show off their best attributes.

However, in many cases, it is popular to leave gems and crystals in a more natural shape. In these cases, the crystals are cut along their existing faces to remove any unattractive and extra bits or to reduce them to a more manageable size. It also often happens that these crystals are only very lightly polished or skip this step completely to achieve a very natural and rugged look. These crystals are called *rough crystals.*

A popular method of shaping and polishing crystals is a process called *tumbling.* Tumbling involves turning larger stones in a rotating barrel full of other, smaller crystals and stones. The smaller stones will begin softening the edges and smoothing the surface of the bigger crystals over time. The stones in which the crystal is rolled are regularly replaced with smaller and finer stones to get an even smoother look and feel. This process brings forth crystals with very interesting and beautiful organic shapes and can last for days, weeks, or even months. The longer the process lasts, the smoother and more rounded the crystal will become.

Crystals can still be bought in their original form, especially in stores specializing in their sales. These ones look quite different from their polished counterparts and can have a very interesting appearance. Crystals that aren't cut or polished are called *raw crystals*.

Chapter 2: The Power of Crystals

Crystals have always had incredible power and have been used as aids in healing and for rituals by hundreds of cultures all around the world. There are many who believe that this power is nothing more than superstitious nonsense, but the fact that the art of crystal healing has spread so far and lasted so long is proof that there is some truth behind the superstition

What Is Crystal Healing?

Crystal healing means to use the unique abilities of different crystals to restore, align, and transform the mind, body, and spirit, as well as to alter or improve natural energy. There are many different ways in which crystals can help you heal and improve your life, and there are hundreds of different crystals to do different things, so much so that you can fill a whole library with all the available knowledge on the subjects. To use healing crystals most effectively, it is best to receive proper training or receive the help of someone who has been properly trained and who has had ample experience using healing crystals. Don't worry, though, because even if you have no training or experience in crystal healing, there are still a lot of things you can do to use crystals to heal and improve yourself and your life. Crystals can also be a very effective first aid tool in emergency situations.

How Does Crystal Healing Work?

Although crystal healing looks, feels, and acts like magic, there is an explanation of how it works. The keywords here are energy, vibration, and resonance. It may not look like it, but everything in this world is made up of energy, including people and crystals. The atoms that form the building blocks of everything vibrate at different frequencies, producing a certain type of energy. The energy within a crystal will react to and resonate with similar types of energy in the world around them, including the energy running through our body. Crystals can help change or improve that energy. The minerals within each will determine the type and frequency of its vibration, giving it its specific properties. Some crystals are good for conducting electricity and light and are used in manufacturing electronics like cellphones, while others are good at transmitting sound and are used for sonar scans and other tasks.

Quartz has an energy that is great for keeping time, and it's always involved in the creation of watches. Healing crystals react to the different energies inside the body. This is why certain types of crystals will have particular effects on a person, such as blue or green stones that tend to be used for healing. Some crystals radiate strong vibrations that affect the energy in the brain, and having these crystals in a room can influence the mood and state of mind of those near to them. A great benefit is that you don't have to be aware of the crystal for it to work, and even if a visitor in your home thinks it's just a decoration, they can still feel the calming effect of the beautiful blue agate displayed on your mantle.

There are many different ways to use crystals, and some methods are more effective with certain types, but all methods can be effective to some extent. It is, however, very important to have an open mind and positive attitude when using crystals to heal, as a negative mindset will influence the energy in your body and cancel out any positive effects the crystals may have. It's perfectly fine to be a little skeptical and unsure, but with an open mind, you may be pleasantly surprised. If you try crystal healing with the thought "this is stupid and it won't work" strongly in your mind, the crystals won't do you any harm, but they probably won't do you any good either.

Colors in Crystal Healing

As mentioned earlier, the minerals that give crystals their color also often give them their specific powers, and so a crystal's effect can be guessed based upon its color. This isn't an exact science, so the rules aren't set in stone, and there are some crystals that defy them, but this color classification can be a good guideline to work with when buying crystals, especially for beginners. It will take a lot of time and effort to memorize the abilities of each individual crystal, even just the basics.

Below are some basic colors and their healing abilities:

- White and colorless crystals tend to encourage peace and purity, meaning they are useful for cleansing the body and spirit and in creating peaceful vibes in an area or around people wearing these types of crystals. They are usually easy to work and connect with and can sometimes be used to help cleanse other crystals or boost their effects. This color association is quite common and has become a strong symbol in many cultures, such as a white wedding dress or white flag. The most common types of white and colorless crystals are clear quartz, opal, fluorite, moonstone, and white opal.

- Blue crystals tend to have calming effects and can help with communication. These types of crystals can make it easier for people to express themselves and communicate with others. They encourage the ability to speak calmly and express ideas and truths, and they are a good tool to aid you in dealing with other people. Lapis lazuli, amazonite, sapphire, turquoise, and topaz are some of the most commonly known types of blue crystals.

- As with the color in general, green crystals represent growth and life, making them perfect for healing. Green crystals can also be used to help develop and nurture new relationships and can keep you focused on your work. Many green crystals also boost fertility. Good examples of green crystals are emerald, malachite, jade, aquamarine, and peridot.

- Pink crystals help boost romantic emotions and attractions and can help in developing and maintaining romantic relationships. They can also encourage more compassion and kindness in a person. The color pink represents love for a reason, after all. Pink crystals can help you overcome heartache and get rid of emotional baggage. These crystals are also believed to be effective against heart diseases. Your most common pink crystal with these abilities is rose quartz, but rhodonite and pink tourmaline are also good examples.

- Yellow crystals are great for helping you feel good and happy. These crystals encourage positive energy, confidence, optimism, enlightenment, and a better understanding of self. They can also help you perceive things differently. They also bring a sense of warmth and joy into your life. Good examples of yellow crystals are labradorite, citrine, and yellow jasper.

- Orange crystals are ideal for artists, as they boost creativity and confidence and encourage freedom of thought. They can also help support and manage big changes in your life and be useful aids when it comes to making decisions. Many reports and studies have shown them to help in dealing with stomach problems. Carnelian, amber, sunstone, and tourmaline all fit into this category.

- Purple crystals are associated with spirituality and mystic energy. They are best suited to help develop the third eye or to simply help you find new inspiration and purpose by tapping into the divine. Purple crystals are often associated with royalty and strong religious figures and were the most often used in magical rituals throughout many cultures. These crystals are great tools to use for deep relaxation or meditation. The most prominent purple crystals are amethyst, spirit quartz, and lepidolite.

- Red crystals tend to be strong and encouraging. They provide energy and passion, help develop courage, and encourage you to take action. They are great for curing apathy and listlessness and can give you a much-needed boost if you are in a negative emotional state. Many red crystals can also speed up your metabolism and help you burn fat a little more quickly. Ruby, red jasper, and garnet are some of the most popular red crystals.

- Brown crystals help garnish stability and inner energy. They assist in keeping you grounded in a busy, chaotic world and can help you regain and maintain your composure. Brown crystals can also help you feel more at ease and comfortable with your surroundings and help you reconnect with the earth and nature. Brown stones can also help treat ADD. Some of the best examples of brown crystals are tiger's eye, smoky quartz, and bronzite

- Black crystals are the guardians of the crystal world, as they provide a sense of security and protect you from negative energy. They tend to alleviate the fear of physical harm, provide mental fortitude, encourage you to keep negative elements out of your life, and help you connect to the physical world. Many black stones can encourage a sense of well being or make you feel more physically powerful and daring, and they are a great comfort to have with you when you are concerned about your physical safety. They also provide additional healing against immune diseases. Black crystals are also often called barrier crystals because of their protective properties. The best known black crystals are onyx, obsidian, jet, and hematite.

There are many other colors to be found in the crystal world, all with their own traits and abilities, but the majority can be divided into one of the basic color groups mentioned above. In some cases, such as with dalmatian jasper, beryl, and certain types of agate, two or more colors are very prominent, and the crystal will usually have a combination of the abilities associated with those colors. These color groupings are a great factor to think about to help decide where to start with buying healing crystals, but if you have the time for it, it is advised to find out a bit more about the properties and abilities of the specific crystals you are buying.

Shapes in Crystal Healing

Different shapes influence the vibrations of crystals, so crystals are often cut into specific forms that can help boost their potency or alter their abilities. Because of this, shapes have taken on certain meanings within the crystal world.

- Spheres are shapes that radiate the energy of a crystal in all directions. They are good for connecting you with your surroundings, in creating balance, and in boosting abilities that encourage peace and relaxation. This shape is also ideal to use for psychic development and can slow down or prevent harmful or imbalanced energies. This shape is considered to be great for helping develop the third eye. Crystals cut into a spherical shape are often great aids in meditation. The sphere is the most common shape used in crystal scrying.

- Pyramids are considered a sacred shape and have been used to harness power by many civilizations throughout history, with ancient Egyptians being a good example. This type of shape harnesses and amplifies energy tremendously, and crystals cut into this shape have very strong effects. If crystals that encourage energy flow and help channel energy are cut into a pyramid shape, they can be a great tool to boost the abilities of other crystals. Pyramids are a good shape to place around the home and can be a good centerpiece for a crystal grid, as it enhances the entire grid.

- Cube shapes often occur naturally among some crystal types, and this shape tends to have a grounding effect; cubic crystals can help ground and seal natural energy. They also root you to physical plain and are a great shape for crystals with physical type abilities.

- Crystal points and towers are a very common shape for crystals and often occur naturally. These shapes are perfect for manifesting energy and intentions, as well as for directing energy. Many crystals that form natural points are only lightly polished and have the bottom cut off to form a base they can stand on.

- Crystal clusters occur when many crystal points grow together on a single matrix. These clusters direct energy in many different directions and vibrate at a much higher frequency, making their abilities stronger than the same amount of individual crystals. Crystal clusters are absolutely great for displaying around the house as they spread large amounts of energy over a large space, and they are very attractive and fascinating to look at. Admiring a large crystal cluster can sometimes keep you busy for ages.

- Heart-shaped crystals help attract love and affection and connect with our hearts. Small hearts are easy to carry with you, while larger hearts can be strategically placed throughout the house, such as in the bedroom. Almost any type of crystal can be cut into a heart shape, but it is especially effective when combined with crystals that boost feelings of love and attraction.

- Crystals can be cut into faceted or rounded wands which are mainly used in crystal massage. The pointed end of the wand is used to direct the energy through your body and aura, while the wider base can help remove negative energy. These crystals can also be utilized to channel other types of energy.

- Tumbled crystals are best for beginners. They have a smooth, organic shape that radiates energy gently, and the rounded edges make them safe and comfortable to keep directly on the body for a long period of time. They tend to be a bit smaller, which makes it easy to keep them in a bag, in the car, in little bowls all around the house, or tucked under a pillow. Another great benefit of tumbled crystals is that it is the cheapest shape for crystals, making it affordable to obtain a wide variety of crystals to experiment with.

- It often happens that crystals are carved into different sculptures that can have great significance. The specific shape is determined by the purpose and can have corresponding effects. Crystals can be carved into religious symbols to help boost spirituality or into specific animal shapes to connect with spirit animals. Crystals cut into yin and yang shapes can help provide balance in life. Crystal skulls are deeply connected to myth and lore and are believed to encourage healing. Many believe that angel-shaped crystals can help you connect to and channel angelic energies. There are hundreds of shapes that crystals can be cut and carved into, each having their own significance and effects.

Crystal Placement

Although placement doesn't have a direct impact on the effects of a crystal, it is important to carefully consider where to put a crystal in your home. Every room in a house has a specific purpose, and the shapes, effects, and abilities of the crystals within a room should mirror that purpose. Crystals with calming effects should be placed in rooms that need peace and quiet, such as a library or study. Crystals that enhance focus and determination are more suitable for workplaces, and crystals that improve communication and provide relaxed and comfortable energy are a great addition to dining and living rooms, where guests are usually entertained.

Having a crystal in the wrong place can have undesirable effects. A good example is placing a crystal that boosts intense emotion and provides energy in a baby's bedroom, when crystals with soothing, relaxing, and protective effects would be a better choice. Another thing to consider carefully when placing crystals is the different types of crystals that might end up sharing the same space. Combining crystals by putting them together or close to each other can be a great way to manage their abilities and effects in a space with more precision, and wonderful things can happen when you have the right crystal combinations. Unfortunately, bad combinations are also a possibility, and the energies in different crystals can clash with one another and have a negative effect, or they can completely cancel each other out and render each other virtually useless.

Chapter 3: Crystals for Everyone

Crystals aren't racist, sexist, religious zealots or biased in any way. Things like age and personality don't matter, and anyone willing to put in the time and effort can try crystal healing. The only prerequisites are an open mind and a very basic understanding of how to apply crystal healing, since simply buying a healing crystal isn't going to change your life. Crystals are fairly easy to come by, and always ready to improve your life. Unfortunately, crystals can be picky at times. Different types of crystal resonate better with different people. A crystal that works miracles for me, may not work for you at all. This is because the energy in a crystal simply doesn't react well to the energy inside your body. This can be a big factor in why many people dismiss crystal healing as a fantasy: they try a very basic recipe for "how to fix a certain problem with this specific crystal" and end up gaining no effects simply because the crystal doesn't resonate with them. There are many crystals with similar effects and abilities, so if one crystal does not work for you, try different crystals with similar properties until you find something that works for you. Choosing a crystal that resonates well with your own energy is especially important when the crystal is meant to be worn for long periods of time, but more on choosing crystals a little later.

Birthstones

This is a system that allocates specific crystals and gemstones to the months of the year. It is a fairly old concept that has undergone some changes, but the current tradition is to give someone a birthstone corresponding with the month they are born in. Birthstones are usually worn as a piece of jewelry, and for many people, birthstones are their first introduction to crystals. Many believe this system found its origins with *Aaron's breastplate*, which is mentioned in the book of Exodus in the bible. This breastplate was studded with twelve gemstones to represent the twelve tribes of Israel, and different interpretations of old texts determined which gemstones these would be, and each was assigned a month of the year. In the eighth and ninth century B.C. the Christian church assigned a stone to each of the twelve apostles, and the custom was to own a set of twelve birthstones and wear each stone during the month assigned to them. This was done in an attempt to honor the apostles and as a teaching method for children to help remember their names. The custom of wearing only the stone assigned to your own month is a much more modern concept that can be dated back to somewhere between the 1500s to the 1800s. These birthstones varied due to different translations and interpretations, but a general pattern could be detected. In 1912, the American National Association of Jewelers put together a standard list of birthstones, which has now become the global standard. There is very little correspondence to historical origins or crystal abilities and symbolism in this list, and many believe this specific list to be little more than a sales pitch. There have been many different cultures around the world that used the birthstone concept, each with their own personal touches. The Chinese culture, as an example, assigns the stones to the twelve zodiac signs rather than the months.

Another system of birthstones uses a color wheel that indicates colors associated with the different time of the year, and associates crystals of the same color to the twelve months. This color wheel system uses a much more accurate approach in terms of symbology, psychology and a study of the use of talismans throughout history to determine which crystal types are more suited to a person based on the time of year they were born in. This system can be a good place to start when you're looking to buy your first healing crystal and want to find something that resonates well with you. Here is a list of the crystal color types that are associated with the different months and some examples:

- 21 Dec to 19 Jan - violet-colored crystals like amethyst, purple agate, and fluorite

- 20 Jan to 18 Feb - indigo-colored crystals like tanzanite, sodalite, and lapis lazuli

- 19 Feb to 19 Mar - blue-colored crystals like aquamarine, blue agate, and kyanite

- 20 Mar to 19 Apr - turquoise-colored crystals like turquoise, and some variants of aquamarine and agate

- 20 Apr to 20 May - green-colored crystals like emerald, alexandrite, and jade

- 21 May to 20 Jun - olive-colored crystals like prehnite and pyromorphite

- 21 Jun to 21 Jul - yellow-colored crystals like citrine, yellow apatite, and cat's eye

- 22 Jul to 21 Aug - gold-colored crystals like golden beryl and cat's eye

- 22 Aug to 22 Sep - orange-colored crystals like amber, carnelian, and sunstone

- 23 Sep to 21 Oct - scarlet-colored crystals like red emerald and red beryl

- 22 Oct to 20 Nov - red-colored crystals like ruby, red jasper, and garnet

- 21 Nov to 20 Dec - amethyst-colored crystals like cacoxenite

Crystal Healing for Children

Any parent will tell you that the question they ask the most is "Is this safe for my child?" In this case, the answer is yes. Crystal healing is perfectly safe for children and should be encouraged, as they are perfect for crystal healing. Children experience the same effects as adults when working with crystals and are naturally more open and susceptible to the energy emitted by crystals, meaning the effects are stronger on them than adults. They are almost always fascinated by crystals and are willing to simply believe in the magic of crystals. This makes crystals even more effective on children and can help bring a sense of awe and wonder into their everyday lives. Practically from birth, children are able to reap the benefits of crystal healing, which can come with some bonuses. There are many crystals that can help make childbirth smoother and easier for both mother and child, and calming crystals can be used in a baby's bedroom to encourage deeper and more restful sleep. Crystals can be used to protect children from nightmares and slightly temper or encourage specific moods, and in the early stages can even be used as a healing tool. Crystals can be great for teaching children colors and shapes, and even counting. Creative little games using crystals can be thought up to stimulate their minds and creativity, all while they receive the wonderful healing energies from handling and being near the crystals. The time spent teaching your child about crystals and playing these little games with them can be a great opportunity to bond with them and develop a good relationship. In less severe situations like light colds or very minor injuries, crystals can be a much more natural alternative to chemical-based remedies. Specific crystals can also be a good way to better manage restlessness and ADD in children. A little later in life, crystals can be a great help for children at school. Having a healing crystal with them at school can children stay focused on their work, improve their skills at making friends, protect them from too much negative energy, and give them a sense of comfort and security. Especially on the first day of school or during important events, the familiar feel of a crystal lying coolly in the palm of their hand can do a lot to help your child ease off some anxiety and feel more reassured and confident.

There are some minor risks involved with introducing children to crystals. Smaller crystals can be a choking hazard for very young children, and sharp points and hard edges can hurt your child. Crystals should be kept far out of the reach of children, and it is advised to start off with round or tumbled crystals that don't have any cutting or poking edges and corners. It is also important to ensure that children aren't allowed to handle crystals without the supervision of a responsible adult until they have proven themselves to be careful and responsible enough to work with crystals on their own.

Crystal Healing for Pets

Just like with children, animals experience the same benefits from crystals. Kind words and a few crystals can help animals heal a lot faster, and their moods and behavior can be managed a little easier. Using crystal healing on animals is a very intuitive process, as they can't communicate their problems as effectively as people, and you usually have to observe the animal and guess whether the crystal is having the right effect or not, but it becomes easier the more you spend time learning how your pet reacts. Crystals can be used to help heal illnesses and minor injuries, ease aches and pains in older animals and, in a worst-case scenario, help ease the passing of a beloved pet when it reaches the end of its life. As always, crystal healing works through proximity and contact, but it can be a little tricky to get a pet to carry one around with them. A good way to ensure a pet always has a crystal with them is to attach it to their collar. Sewing crystals into favorite toys or placing them around their favorite sleeping spots are another way to ensure that pets spend a lot of time near healing crystals. For birds and hamsters, it's a good idea to attach crystals to the outside of their cages. Many of the common techniques of crystal healing such as crystal massages and water infusions, which will be discussed in detail in the next chapter, are effective for pets too. In many cases, such as with a massage, pets will even enjoy the healing process a lot.

Chapter 4: Healing with Crystals

Simply owning a few healing crystals and wearing them from time to time isn't going to change your life. Just like with everything else, crystal healing takes some time and a little bit of effort. It isn't much, but you do need to put in some work. But the results are well worth it. There are so many ways in which crystals can improve your life.

Crystals and Chakras

Chakras are a very important part of life, especially when it comes to energy, and so, understanding how chakras work will always be a requirement for proper crystal healing.

What Are Chakras?

Like blood, energy flows throughout the entire body. It travels along set pathways and circulates in a single direction. This energy plays an important role in the health of your mind, body, and spirit. Irregularities in the flow of energy can have severe consequences, and it is important to keep the flow as steady as possible. Throughout the body, there are seven main energy centers throughout the body called chakras. These chakras send your energy throughout the rest of your body and manage the balance and flow of your energy. They act almost like gateways, opening and closing to limit the amount of energy allowed through. The first of the seven chakras is found at the base of the spine and run in a line to the crown of the head. Each chakra has its own function and represents important elements of life. Each chakra also has a color assigned to it that represents its purpose and the type of energy it works with.

The first chakra is called the root chakra, or Muladhara. It sits at the very base of your spine, near your tailbone. The purpose of this chakra is to ground you by connecting all your energy to the earth. It creates stability and is responsible for everything you need to survive from day to day. This chakra is associated with the color red. The most common signs of a balanced root chakra are a sense of accomplishment when thinking about elements such as safety and financial stability, and a strong feeling of being connected to your human experience. An overactive root chakra can cause unease, jitteriness, paranoia, digestive problems, hip pain, and lower back issues. An underactive chakra can sap your concentration and prevent your thoughts from staying grounded in the moment. The most easily recognizable sign is an unhealthy amount of daydreaming.

The second chakra is called the sacral chakra, also known as Svadhishana. This chakra is located just below the belly button and is focused on the self. This chakra is centered around your identity as a human being living on this earth, here and now. It encourages you to enjoy and appreciate the fruits of your hard labor and provides creative energy. The sacral chakra helps you enjoy life and is connected to the color orange. A balanced chakra will help you find more pleasure in the good things in life, but also avoid overdoing them. It will be easier for you to find inspiration in things like good food, intimacy and creative activities and you will feel good about and satisfied by them. An overactive sacral chakra can cause gluttony, obesity, hormone imbalances and addiction. An underactive chakra may lead to impotence, depression, and a devastating lack of creativity and passion.

Third is the solar plexus chakra, or Manipura. It is located at the center of your belly button and is the source of your self-confidence, personal power, and identity as an individual. This is where your "gut-feelings" come from when you instinctively know a person, location, or situation just isn't right for you. The solar plexus chakra is connected to the color yellow and helps you feel empowered, wiser, more decisive and more confident in who you are. It is often called the warrior chakra, as a perfectly balanced chakra creates the same feeling as a warrior going into battle, confident in his ability to win and wise enough to understand what he is fighting for. An overactive solar plexus chakra can lead to a short temper, greed, a lack of empathy and sympathy, and a strong need to micromanage and be in control at all times. It can also lead to issues with your digestive system and severe problems with your internal organs. An underactive solar plexus chakra can cause indecision, insecurity, a lack of energy and a tendency to be needy.

Your heart chakra - or Anahata - is next. It is located in your chest directly over your heart. It deals with strong emotions and especially love for both yourself and others. It is also strongly associated with growth and healing, which is why it is represented by the color green. It can help you see the goodness and compassion in others during tough times and allows you to love and appreciate yourself and other people in equal measures. An overactive heart chakra can cause you to always prioritize the needs of others above your own to an unhealthy extent. It can cause serious problems in your relationship with yourself and often leads to palpitations, an increased heart rate and heartburn. If your heart chakra is underactive, it can close you off from others and prevent you from building deep relationships. You can feel disconnected from your body and suffer from circulation problems as well.

The fifth chakra is the throat chakra, also called Vishuddha. This one sits right in the center of your collarbone and empowers communication and lets you speak your personal truths with clarity and confidence. It is just above your heart chakra and is thus also connected to love and compassion. The throat chakra lets you speak more easily from the heart. It helps you find the right words to carry your message over and to inspire those around you. It is associated with the color blue. If your throat chakra is overactive, you will often be accused of having a loud voice, and you will have a tendency to interrupt others. It may also be possible that you love to hear yourself talk a little too much. An overactive throat chakra can cause a sore throat, mouth ulcers, cavities, and frequent throat infections. If your throat chakra is underactive, you probably have trouble raising your voice and expressing yourself. You act shy around others or pull yourself away from conversations completely. Because unused energy from the throat chakra is usually diverted to the third chakra, an underactive throat chakra can cause digestive problems.

Directly between your eyebrows, you can find your sixth chakra, called the third eye chakra, or Anja. This chakra is associated with psychic powers, as it deals with information beyond the five senses. The sixth chakra helps you find balance and peace with both the material and physical worlds and can help you maintain your faith. It is also the source of good intuition. The third eye chakra is represented by the color purple, though some charts use the color indigo as representation, and it is believed that psychic abilities are developed through this chakra. An overactive third eye chakra is incredibly rare, but in such cases, those with an overactive chakra will find their lives consumed and overwhelmed by paranormal experiences and psychic actions like astrology and tarot reading, that distract them from enjoying the human experience. An underactive third eye chakra is much more common and afflicts the majority of people in the world. An underactive sixth chakra completely cuts you off from all psychic energy and prevents you from receiving any information that does not come from the five senses.

Last is the crown chakra, which is called Sahaswana. It is difficult to explain, but this chakra connects you to the universe and the world around you. The crown chakra is placed at the very top of your head, and your consciousness is hidden somewhere in this chakra. Achieving a balanced crown chakra is extremely difficult, and is similar to the Buddhist concept of reaching nirvana, and is the ultimate goal for all spiritual questors and warriors. This chakra is associated with white, or with clear chakras. Many charts use a dark purple to represent this chakra, as white can be difficult to work with. It is impossible to have an overactive crown chakra, and there is nothing wrong with you if your crown chakra is underused. It just means that you are human.

There are many different ways to throw off the balance within your chakras. From using a chakra too much or too little, to blocking it completely, disrupting the natural flow of the energy coming from your chakras can greatly impact your wellbeing, as well as how you walk through life. It is critical to keep your chakras as healthy and balanced as possible if you want the best life has to offer.

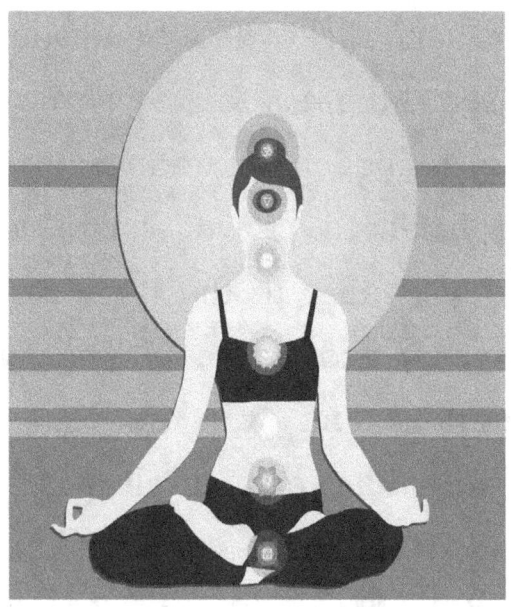

How Crystal Healing Can Help Your Chakras

Chakras provide and control the energy flowing through your body, and crystal healing works through crystals resonating with your natural energy, giving boosts to some types, negating or dampening others, or completely changing how your energy flows and affects you. Thinking like this, it's only natural that crystal healing and chakras go together. Crystals can be a large tool in balancing, cleansing, aligning and unblocking your chakras, as they can help regulate, boost and support the energy of the chakras. Of course, you can't just take any random crystal and start healing. You need to select your stones carefully for each chakra. Luckily there are two simple methods to do that. The first is to choose by purpose and function. Look at the function and purpose of each chakra and choose a crystal with effects that will encourage or boost that purpose, like an amethyst, which boosts spirituality and opens you to the world around you, for your third eye chakra, and malachite, a strong healing crystal, or rose quartz, a crystal that encourages love and affection, for your heart chakra. A crystal with an effect that supports the purpose of the chakra you want to use it with will help strengthen that energy and maintain and continuous flow of that type of energy throughout the body. Another, even easier way, is to choose by color. Looking back a little, you might notice that the general functions and abilities of the different colors of crystals correspond to the functions of the chakra of the same color. Blue crystals help with communication, green crystals heal, and white and clear crystals channel energy and encourage purity. In correspondence, the throat chakra deals with communication and expressing yourself, and is represented with blue; the heart chakra is green, and is the chakra of love, hope, and healing; and the crown chakra is represented by white and is all about connecting to the energy of the world around you. Choosing stones by the colors of your chakras is the quickest and simplest way to choose which crystals to use for healing your chakras. Many crystal stores sell sets of seven crystals that match the colors of the seven chakras called *chakra stones*. These sets are selected and put together specifically to be used for cleansing and aligning your chakras and are especially useful for beginners.

Now that you know which crystals to use, it's time to learn how to use them. As always, contact and proximity are how this works. Carrying your chakra stones with you is a good idea to get a steady flow of healing energy from them. If you're having trouble with a specific chakra, wear a crystal to help cleanse and strengthen it on you at all times, either in a pocket or purse or as a piece of jewelry. This is a simple way to give basic support to your chakras, but taking the time to have a full healing session can have a much stronger effect. Find somewhere calm and quiet where you can be comfortable and lie down on a soft blanket or carpet. Lie on your back and take a few deep breaths to get calm and relaxed. Place your crystals on your body directly where the chakras are located - the crystal for the crown chakra should be placed on the ground directly above your head, and the root chakra on the ground between your legs.lie there for ten to twenty minutes and let the crystals do their work. Clear your mind and focus on your breathing, or on your chakras and the crystals. Move your thoughts from one chakra to the next and feel the energy flowing through them. Visualize each chakra as a colored wheel of energy turning in a clockwise direction. Let your worries and problems go for a while and let in the healing. After a session like this, you should feel more centered, balanced and relaxed. This method can be used to heal only a few specific chakras, or even just one if it's giving you some serious problems. Just holding a chakra stone near or over your chakra and focusing on its energy can be an easy way to get some quick healing done in a pinch.

It's important to clear your crystals or chakra stones before and after using them to align and balance your chakras. A crystal filled with negative or unwanted energy won't be able to do much to heal your chakras and might throw off its balance even more. You should also make sure your crystals are properly charged, especially the ones you wear as jewelry or carry with you wherever you go. The more you use a crystal, the quicker it loses its energy.

Crystal Healing and Meditation

Meditation is a method of focusing the mind and turning off unnecessary mental chatter. It helps you focus your mind on one specific thought, action, activity or intention. Meditating can help you remove stress from your life, lower your blood pressure and improve spiritual growth. Meditation can also help improve your crystal healing. Meditating on a crystal can help you better connect with its energy and learn to understand it better. Meditation can help you become more in tune with your crystals, and it's a good idea to spend some time meditating with every one of your crystals every now and then. This can help you understand how they work and feel their effects on you much more acutely. You can even have what some call a *crystal day,* where you spend the whole day meditating with crystals, starting with crystals that have a strong energizing effect. These are usually your red crystals. Move on to orange and yellow and green, working your way through the rainbow until you go from violet to white and finally to clear crystals. This can be an incredible experience that can bring you in tune with the highest possible frequency of crystal vibration and may leave you feeling energized, exalted, and blissed out. It might be a good idea to meditate with a black or brown crystal afterward to ground yourself again. Here is a good exercise to help you meditate with a crystal:

Find a calm, comfortable place where you won't be interrupted, especially by your phone and other people, or distracted by unnecessary things. Again, your phone can be a problem. In fact, just turn off your phone and leave it on the opposite side of your home when you meditate. To start, get yourself settled in a comfortable sitting position and set up your crystal. You can either put it on the floor or a low table in front of you or hold it with both hands in your lap. Focus on your breathing while you let go of all your anxiety and tension. Take a deep breath, making sure that the exhale is just a little longer than the exhale. Breathe in positive and relaxing energy and breathe out all the negativity you have bottled up inside. Keep this up until you've established a slow, steady rhythm. Now shift your focus to your crystal. See its color and shape and feel its weight if you have it in your hands. Feel its vibrations running through you as you study the finer points of the crystal. All the lines and speckles of color. The inner planes and little flaws that make this crystal unique. When you feel you're ready to move on, close your eyes and begin contemplating your crystal. Focus your thoughts on the energy moving into you from the crystal, and let the crystal teach you what it wants you to know about it. This step can be as long or short as you need it to be. When you're finished with your meditation, you can open your eyes again. Plant your feet firmly on the ground and give yourself some time to come back to the present and your body again. Holding a grounding crystal like a smoky quartz or boji stone can help with that.

On the other hand, crystals can help improve your meditation in general. If you're having trouble focusing your mind on the subject of your meditation, having a suitable crystal on you or in the room with you can help focus your mind on where it needs to be. You can either use crystals that improve concentration in general, or you can use a crystal related to what you are meditating on, like using stones like amethyst or lepidolite to assist you when you're meditating for religious reasons or to strengthen your third eye. Or using green crystals when your meditation focuses on healing and growth.

Whether your meditation is focused on your crystals or you're using crystals to enhance your meditation, it's very important to make sure that your crystals are always properly cleansed and have pure energy. Impure energy in a crystal can disrupt your meditation have the opposite effect if you're not careful.

Using Crystals to Improve Your Life

Improving the quality of your life is what crystal healing is all about. From improving your mood to controlling certain elements in your life daily to encourage healing and improving mental stability, there's a crystal that can do it for you, and there are different ways to use these crystals according to what you need.

Combining Crystals and Crystal Healing

Before we get to the various methods of practicing crystal healing, it might be good to know that you can combine crystals with each other for different results. Many crystals have abilities that complement or counter one another, and one crystal likely won't be enough to get all the results out of your crystal healing. Say, for instance, you're having trouble developing your relationship on an emotional level, you could use a rose quartz to boost feelings of love and attraction, and then add an amethyst to dampen the intense physical attraction and raising it to a more spiritual level. Adding a clear quartz to the mix will increase the strength of the impact the crystals have.

Combining different shapes and sizes can help you further narrow down your precise results, as the shape of your crystals have their own effects, and larger crystals have more energy to give than smaller ones.

A wonderful thing about crystal healing is that you can also use it together with other types of healing, medicines, and therapies. Crystals can greatly help improve the results of these healing techniques, and vice versa. Adding essential oils to a crystal massage can do wonders for the mind, body, and spirit.

Wearing Crystals

Wearing crystals is the simplest and most common way of using crystal healing. Crystals emit their own energy constantly, as well as repel and remove other types of energy. By keeping a crystal on your body or in your pocket, that crystal will continue resonating with your energy and you will feel its effects as long as you have it with you. Putting on a crystal necklace or having tumbled stone in your pocket can be compared to taking a vitamin in the morning to nourish you throughout the whole day. Crystal shapes can easily be used to determine exactly what you want to do with your crystal healing, and it's very simple to combine crystals if you want to. The biggest limitation of this method is the size of the crystal. It could become quite tricky to carry a crystal in your coat pocket or tuck it into your bra if it's the size of a tennis ball. Because these crystals tend to be used long term, it's important to regularly clear and charge your crystals to gain the best benefits from them.

Placing Crystals on Your Body

This is the method you use when you want to do something very specific right now. Place your crystal directly where you want its abilities to affect you. This will direct the energy of the crystal directly to the area it's in contact with, and you will feel its effect the strongest in that spot. This method works exactly like applying a balm to a burn or ice to a swollen wrist or ankle. If you feel nauseous, hold a piece of sodalite to your stomach, or if you have a headache, sit down for a while and press a quartz on the spot where the pain is the strongest.

Placing Crystals Around the House

Your home is a very important part of your life, and using crystals is a great way to make your living space a place of safety, serenity, and healing. You can set the charge and mood for each room, helping you build a more perfect home for yourself. You can place barrier crystals at your doors and windows to ward off negative energy and protect your health. Scatter calming and healing crystals around your bathroom to make those long, relaxing baths even better. Put pink crystals in your bedroom to attract romantic energy.

Crystal shapes strongly into play here, as the shape of the crystal can help regulate how the crystal affects the feeling of the room. For example, if you have guests coming over for dinner, us a large round amazonite crystal as a centerpiece. Its ability to encourage communication and truth will be spread evenly all over the room. Scatter a few pieces of tumbled malachite and fluorite around the amazonite to gently radiate a sense of confidence and calmness. Not only will this make a beautiful display and an interesting conversation piece, but it will also help your guests feel confident and relaxed around each other and help them communicate with one another truthfully and with ease.

The same concept can be applied to your car. Simply put a crystal or two, or three or four, on your dashboard, the backseat, the glove compartment, or even the cupholders, and you can receive healing and protection from your crystals as you drive to work or do your shopping.

Sleeping with Crystals

Just because your conscious mind turns off and stops working, doesn't mean your crystals do. There is no reason why you can't receive some crystal healing while you sleep. In fact, it might be even better than when you're awake. When sleeping, your subconscious takes over and you become more susceptible to a crystal's energy. Placing crystals near your bed can help you heal at an accelerated pace while you sleep. They can help you relax before going to bed and protect you from bad dreams and encourage good ones. You should consider which crystals you use carefully. Crystals that improve communication will do you little good in your sleep, and crystals that invigorate you aren't a good idea, but tucking a calming crystal under your pillow can be a great way to fight insomnia.

Crystal Grids

Crystal grids are all about combining crystals and using shapes. Crystal grids are built by placing crystals in a specific geometric shape that has been predetermined. Learning all the different types of grids and how to use them can take a long time, but most are willing to put in the hours, as crystal grids are a very powerful tool. Crystal grids are used to strengthen intention, manifest ambition and greatly enhance the abilities of your crystals. These grids are designed to create especially effective combinations, and the sacred geometries used make your crystals much stronger than they would normally be individually. Crystal grids are also commonly used to enhance spells and form a part of rituals in many cultures and religions. All crystal grids have a larger stone in the center that forms the core of the grid. These are usually pyramids or points to direct and manifest the power, but other shapes can also be used, depending on the purpose of your grid. Next are tumbled and rough stones to form the rest of the grid, and a clear quartz to connect the crystals and activate the grid. Building a grid can be easy to build, but they require a flat surface with enough space for the entire grid. These grids should remain undisturbed, so if you have a cat or a small child, it is important to find a way to keep your grid safe from them. Here are instructions to build a basic crystal grid:

1. Start with your intention. Decide what you want to do with this grid, and build up from that. You can write down your intention on a piece of paper and leave it folded on the table, or you can just keep it strongly in your thoughts.

2. Choose a sacred geometry that compliments your intention, as well as all the crystals you are going to use. The crystals should match your intention as much as possible. If you want, you

can build your grid on a board and use wire to fix the crystals in place. This can help you keep the crystals on the grid from accidentally being nudged out of place, and you can even have it framed when you're done.

3. Lay out your crystals according to the grid, starting with the outside and working your way towards the center. Your focal crystal in the middle of the grid should be placed last. Make sure to keep your mind focused on your intention while you work.

4. Use your clear quartz to connect the points of your grid, again working from the outside inward. Pass your quartz crystal over every single crystal in the grid and keep focussing on your intention.

5. The final step is to make sure your grid won't be disturbed or disrupted, and feel its powerful effect.

Moving Crystals Around the Body

Crystals don't need to stay in the same place for a long time to make them work. Moving crystals around your body can help spread their energy throughout your body or direct their energy flow more accurately. Removing tension and negative energy all around your body can be very easy with this method. You can move the crystals to where they are needed most, and when they've done their healing work there, you can move on to the next troublesome spot. Wands are a good tool to use here and help direct your energy better and can direct precisely where the energy needs to go or needs to be removed from. Moving the crystals through the air around you can help you cleanse your aura and the energy flowing all around you.

A good example of this method is a crystal massage. This is a technique similar to a hot rock massage, but rather than regular heated stones, different types and shapes of crystals are used. These crystals are chosen according to what you want out of the massage, and different types and shapes are used on the different parts of the body. It's possible to get a full body massage or to focus on a specific area. A crystal massage can be an incredible, divine experience, and, if done right, one single crystal massage can achieve results in one session what might require several sessions of regular massage. Crystal massages can be a great way to achieve perfect balance in the mind, body, and spirit. With a little bit of searching, you can find a professional practitioner to give you one of these massages, but the world is also full of courses and books that can teach you to do this yourself - or to teach a friend how to give you a crystal massage.

It is, of course, important to properly clear your crystals before and after using this method.

Water Infusion

Infusing your drinking water with a crystal's healing energy is a good way to heal and cleanse your body from the inside. Water is good for the body and can carry those healing energies throughout your entire body. Filtering your water through healing stones is a good way to infuse your water, or you could let your water stand for a while with a crystal or two in the glass. You should remove the stones from the glass to prevent accidentally swallowing or choking on a stone. A useful product that is fairly new to the market is a water bottle with a chamber at the bottom where you can lock a healing crystal in place. A more common alternative is to use a water bottle with a built-in infuser usually meant for fruits or herbs. You can freely pick and choose which crystals to use, but be careful around crystals like malachite that are made up of toxic minerals. When infusing your water, it is vital that your crystals are clean of any dirt or bacteria before you use them. Cleansing their energy beforehand is also advised.

Chapter 5: Your Own Collection

Now that you understand how crystals work and how to use them properly, it's time to start building your own private, and very personal, collection of healing crystals. This entails a little more than just walking into the first store you see and buying whatever takes your fancy. Buying crystals takes time, attention and careful consideration. This entire chapter is dedicated to helping you choose the right crystals and to teach you how to take care of them.

Choosing the Right Crystals

The first thing you need to do when buying a crystal is to decide what you want it to do. Buying a crystal with a specific purpose in mind is a much better idea than simply choosing a crystal for the sake of owning one. You have an idea of which types of crystal have the right abilities, so keeping your mind focused on what you want to do with the crystal, walk through the store and let your intuition choose for you. Don't think about it. Feel it. A specific crystal might catch your eye for no specific reason, or you might feel one of the crystals pulling at you. That is a good indication that that is the crystal for you. Hold the crystal in your hand and focus your energy on it. You should feel something from it, like sensations of hot or cold, pulsations, or simply just a sense of rightness. If this is the case, you've found your crystal. If you don't feel anything from the crystal you've selected, your search continues. Spotting a crystal through this sense can be difficult at first, but it becomes easier with practice. Sometimes it's simply the color of the crystal or an interesting shape that draws your attention, and that's okay. The crystal chooses you as much as you choose it. Just listen to your instincts and you shouldn't have a problem. Beyond crystals won't work for you, there are even crystals that will work against you. There is nothing wrong with you or the crystal. It just means that the energy in your body vibrates at a frequency that clashes with that of the crystal. Owning a crystal like this can have a very negative influence on your crystal healing process, but a simple way to see if a crystal will reject you is to close your hand around the crystal and hold it against your stomach. Close your eyes and focus on the crystal. You'll definitely feel the crystal pushing against you, trying to get away from your energy. In many cases, you can even see the crystal pushing your body away slightly if the clash is strong enough.

Basic Crystals for Beginners

If you're a beginner, it can be very difficult to know which crystal to buy, especially if you're trying crystal healing out for the first time and you don't have any idea about what to expect or what you want to do with your crystals. Crystal healing might not be for you, and you don't want to end up spending a fortune on a large variety of crystals to experiment with in the hopes that one or two might work for you. To prevent that, here is a list of a few simple, strong crystals that are easy to come by, inexpensive, and bound to tell you if crystal healing is meant for you.

- Clear quartz, which amplifies the effects of your other crystals and amplifies your intention. It is often called the *Master Healer* because it can be used for almost any purpose.

- Amethyst, which is a strong spiritual stone and can be used as a stress reliever or to help in your meditation. Amethyst is a great crystal to have with you in difficult times when you need to look deep into yourself for answers, or when you need an emotional and spiritual boost.

- Tiger's eye carries strong earth energies, making it great for grounding yourself and helping you make logical decisions. It also channels creative energy and can help you get rid of writer's block.

- Bloodstone is a crystal that helps boost the immune system, boosts energy, causes relief for chronic diseases and clears the body of disease and toxins. This stone is well known as the healing crystal, and it's a great aid for athletes.

- Carnelian encourages confidence and motivation. It also awakens passion and attractions and can be used to enhance your sexual experience.

- Smoky quartz is another earth stone that grounds you. It is also great for cleansing your other crystals and the energy in a space, as it draws out negative energy quite well. Smoky quartz is good for relieving panic attacks, negative emotions, and negative memories.

- Hematite is a good barrier stone that provides mental and emotional stability. It encourages blood circulation and draws toxic energy out of your body. Because hematite assists memory function and gives you mental clarity, it's a good stone to keep around when studying.

Where to Buy Crystals

Finding the right place to buy your crystals takes a little homework. Not all stores sell crystals, and specialized crystal stores that sell a large variety and can properly cater to your needs are much less common than we would like. Furthermore, not all stores that sell crystals can be trusted. Many jewelry stores and pharmacies will sell crystal jewelry and birthstones that look authentic enough at first glance but are as often as not nothing more than colored glass. This isn't necessarily an evil plot to sucker you out of your money, but simply a good way to sell more items meant as decorations rather than healing tools. Any healing effects gained from these crystals are a result of the placebo effect, where your mind convinces your body that the crystals are working. Not all of these types of crystals are necessarily fake, mind you, and if you can verify that they are the real deal, you can buy as many of these crystals as you want.

The best place to buy crystals is at a store that specializes in selling them. Because crystals for the purpose of crystal healing aren't a global franchise, these stores tend to be small and tucked into odd corners of the world. These stores can even be businesses run out of the owner's home. In any case, the chances of finding a specialized store in your local mall aren't all that big. Do some research to find a crystal shop in your area, and see if there are any reviews on the place before you take the trip. If you're just moving around town, it won't be hard to recognize one of these stores. A good trademark is a display window filled with crystals of all shapes and sizes, ranging from small carved figures to clusters of raw crystals large enough to cover your hand. Even if they are perfectly organized, shops like these tend to have an organic, natural feel to them, and if you've ever worked with crystal healing before, you should be able to feel something of the energy of the crystals the second you pass through the door.

Shopping online is also a viable option, especially if you don't have a crystal store in your area. Online suppliers often have a very large variety, and it's possible to see what they can get their hands on for you, even if they don't have the supplies on hand. Again, shopping at sites that specialise in crystals and related products is better than general places that sell a bit of everything. Still, a word of caution: not all websites out there are trustworthy. Be careful where you give out your personal information, and don't jump the gun on this one. Do your homework on the sites you visit, and make sure they aren't trying to scam you. Just by scrolling through a few of their pages can easily tell you if they know what they're talking about, and if a site is popular with a lot of frequent customers, it's a good sign that it is trustworthy and provides good services and products. Reading as many reviews given to these websites as possible is also a good way to learn what you can expect from them. The biggest setback of shopping online is that you can't be there to choose your crystal in person and feel its energy. This makes finding the ideal crystal for you harder, but you can still go far with this form of shopping.

How to Spot a Fake

If you're at all interested in crystal healing it is critical that you know the difference between a real and a fake crystal. Fake crystals can do a great deal for you if you just want a nice piece of jewelry or a decoration for your home, but no matter how beautiful they are, these cut and colored piece of glass, resin or plastic have no helpful energy or healing properties. Another type of fake is when your cheaper, more common types of crystals are dyed to resemble rarer and more expensive crystals. The surest way to detect if a crystal is a fake or not is through a series of scientific tests, but trying to do that in a store is a little ridiculous. Here are some simple tips for discovering a fake on sight.

- To detect the difference between clear quartz and glass or resin, look for bubbles. Real quartz crystals may have flaws inside, but they do not have small, perfectly round bubbles.

- Look for flaws. Crystals are not perfect, and that is where their beauty lies. If a line in a crystal is too regular and the same thickness all around, they may be glass. If the color is too perfect and solid, it's most likely dyed. Transparent and translucent crystals have interesting little flaws on the inside that can be hard to recreate.

- With crystal points, look at the symmetry. If a crystal point is unusually symmetrical, it isn't natural. It was cut that way.

- Hold transparent and very translucent crystals against a piece of paper or card with some writing on it. Real crystals won't magnify the letters, and some may even blur the letters a little. Glass crystals tend to magnify letters.

- Check the color. If a crystal has an unnaturally bright, rich or neon color to it, it is likely that the crystals have been dyed or treated.

- Check the base of the crystal for paint or glue. It often happens that the base of a crystal is painted to make its color look richer, and crystal clusters might be a bunch of rocks glued together.

- Ask the seller. In some cases fake crystals aren't there because the seller wants to cheat you, but because they know some people just want something pretty. They will most likely be more than happy to tell you if there are any fake crystals or crystals that have been dyed.

- Check for extremely deep cracks. It often happens that small crystal chunks that normally aren't useable are ground into a fine powder. This powder is poured into a mold and compressed to form a new, larger crystal. These crystals tend to have deep cracks.

- Check for excess dye in the cracks of a crystal.

- Check the price. If a rare or normally expensive crystal us unexpectedly cheap, chances are it isn't real.

- Try to find out if the seller is a trustworthy supplier by asking around about them and looking them up. Reviews are a good way to find out more about the supplier.

- Know your crystals. Before buying crystals, do a bit of research on the crystals you are interested in buying to find out their typical colors, shape, rarity and price range. This can do a lot to help you detect some obvious fakes in a store.

These tips can help you a great deal, but some fakes are very well made, and many of these won't do you much good when you're shopping online, but there are some easy ways to test for a fake crystal at home.

- Give the crystals a good wash. In many cases, the dye on a crystal will wash right off.

- Press the tip of a hot needle against your crystal. This may not be very effective against glass, as it will react the same as real crystals, but it can help against other fakes. A real crystal will simply form a small scorch mark that you can remove easily enough, but plastic, resin, and compressed crystals will begin to melt.

- If the crystal is soft enough, make a small cut with a metal knife. Under a magnifying glass, a real crystal will have jagged edges around the cut while glass or resin will have smooth edges. You can also make a small cut to see if there is a different color under a layer of strong dye.

- With some crystals, like turquoise, you can use UV lighting to detect a fake or dyed crystal. It will take a little bit of research to find out which crystals will have a blacklight effect and which won't, but it's well worth the effort.

To help you look out for counterfeiting a little better, here is a list of crystals that are most commonly faked, dyed or treated:

- Agate

- Carnelian

- Citrine

- Clear quartz

- Lapis lazuli

- Purple and pink jade

- Smoky quartz

- Turquoise

There are some cases where crystals are treated or faked where it is a feature and not a dishonest practice. A good example Swiss blue- and London blue topaz, where a regular blue topaz is treated to give it these intense hues. Opalite is another good example. Opal is very rare in gem form and usually very expensive, but it is a very beautiful stone that plays with light and color in incredible ways. Opalite is a special type of glass that is treated to recreate these effects. Opalite can be cut and polished into various shapes and is popular as jewelry. In cases like these, it is a given that the crystals and gemstones are not natural, but many sellers will still explain this to you to make sure you understand. The prices of these crystals will also be made accordingly.

Something to consider is that while paying dearly for a turquoise, only to discover it's dyed howlite is unforgivable, not all fakes are necessarily bad. Compressed crystals may not be made of one solid rock, but they often still have the same healing properties if they aren't dyed to pose as more expensive crystals. Treated crystals may also do what you want them to do. As an example, citrine is a very rare crystal and it usually has a white wine or pale yellow color. In most cases, amethyst is treated with heat until it turns orange and is sold as citrine. This may not be too bad, as amethyst has properties and abilities very similar to citrine, and many people prefer the brighter, more vibrant stone in their jewelry. In this case, you have a fully functioning, beautifully colored crystal at a fraction of what you would normally pay for a real citrine. Dye isn't always too horrible either. Where is the harm in a blue lace agate that has had its color enhanced a little? The dye won't diminish its ability to heal. There are even synthetic crystals created in laboratories using the exact same methods and ingredients as their naturally grown counterparts, just a lot less time. These crystals are still basically the same thing. Even though it is very frustrating and disappointing when you buy a crystal, only to discover that it's a fake and you've been tricked out of your money, this isn't always the case with fake crystals. If the seller is open and honest with you about the fakes, you understand where you stand with these fakes and are still willing to pay a fair and reasonable price for what you get, there is no reason why you can't be satisfied with any of your crystals.

After Buying

Once you've bought your crystal, it's time to make it yours. The first thing you need to do is clear your crystal of all negative energy or the energy of everyone who touched the crystal before you. There are many different ways to cleanse a crystal, which will be discussed soon, and you should choose what works for you. You can then give your crystal a little more purpose by setting your intentions. This is often called *programming*. As mentioned above, it's better to buy a crystal with a purpose in mind, and programming is basically confirming that purpose with your crystal and filling it with your own energy and vibrations. This way it will be able to resonate better with you and give you the best results. Programming crystals isn't limiting your crystal to one purpose alone or telling it how to heal you, but telling it where you need its help the most. Like going to a doctor and telling them you have a sore throat. That way the doctor knows what to look for and where to start. Crystal programming is an option and not a necessity. It may be a good help for crystals you're carrying with you or using long term, you don't have to program a crystal if you don't feel it's necessary. If you want to, however, here is how it's done.

1. Find a quiet place where you won't be disturbed or interrupted.

2. Take your crystal in both hands and hold it at the same level as your third eye chakra.

3. Close your eyes, take a few deep breaths to find inner calm, focus on your crystal and your specific intention for it.

4. Either silently in your head or out loud, tell the crystal what you want it to do. You can ask however you're comfortable with, but some examples could help.

"I program this crystal to help me improve my relationship."

"I charge this crystal with the intention to strengthen my resolve and work ethic."

"Crystal, I ask you to help me by healing my aches and pains from this illness."

Again, it is important to do what works for you personally, and if you don't feel comfortable programming your crystal, you shouldn't force yourself to do it.

Caring for Your Collection

Like any healing implements, your healing crystals require care and maintenance to keep them working properly. No medical professional would dream of using a dirty scalpel or malfunctioning defibrillator. In the same way, you shouldn't use crystals that have lost their charge or are cluttered with unwanted and negative energy. There are three main parts to keeping your crystals at their best: cleaning, clearing, and charging.

Cleaning Crystals

No one likes a dirty crystal, and dust, grime and all manner of other forms of dirt can interfere with the energy of your crystal. Crystals that are used in direct contact with your body or to infuse water need to be cleaned very thoroughly to prevent harmful bacteria and diseases. For large display crystals, a frequent good dusting ought to be enough, but with carved crystals or crystal clusters, it will take a little more work to clean up the nooks and crannies that just love gathering dust. The simplest way to clean a crystal is by rinsing it off with water and washing it with a soft cloth. Unfortunately, some crystals like azurite, selenite, angelite, and phenakate will begin to dissolve in water, and they should be kept well away. In these cases, you should use a clean, dry cloth to rub the dirt away. When cleaning crystals, you should make sure your cloth is soft and won't shed any fibers. A good alternative is using an otherwise unused, soft-bristled toothbrush to clean your crystals. When handling your crystals, keep in mind how rough you are. Some crystals can take a bit of rough handling without any problems, but there are many types of crystals that are softer and tend to scratch or break if you aren't careful. You should be especially careful and gentle with crystal clusters that have small crystals connected to the grid by only a very small area.

Cleansing Crystals

This refers to clearing and cleaning the energy of your crystal and restoring it to its natural state. Crystals have a tendency to absorb energy from the world around them, including from other people. If people touch your crystals, it will automatically absorb their energy, which usually doesn't work well with your own. This could cause problems with the crystal's ability to resonate with your energy and heal you, and this is why you shouldn't have anyone else touching your crystals. Crystals will also absorb negative energy in the air that you don't want to be sent your way. Crystals used in healing sessions or to draw out and ward off negative energy are especially problematic in this regard. Crystals should be cleansed frequently to remove all this unwanted energy and make their energy pure and clean again. There are many different ways to cleanse a crystal. Some methods don't work well with certain types, and some can be more difficult to come by depending on time and place, but there are enough different methods for you to find something that works perfectly for you.

- Water is a great way to cleanse your crystals. Find a source of natural water like a pond, lake, river, spring or waterfall, and hold your crystal in the water for a while to let the clean water wash away the negative energy. You can even leave your crystal outside in the rain for a good cleansing. Leaving your crystal out a little longer during a thunderstorm can even help you charge your crystal with new energy. Of course, you shouldn't use this method on crystals that dissolve in water.

- Placing your crystals in saltwater for a few hours can also cleanse them, as the salt will help the water draw out and absorb the negative energy. Again, water isn't meant for all crystals, and you shouldn't use this method on crystals with a hardness lower than seven, as the salt can scratch and damage crystals that are too soft.

- The earth is a great cleanser, and you can harness this natural power by burying your crystals in the ground for about four hours or so. This is an especially strong method to use on earthy and grounding crystals like smoky quartz and tiger's eye. If you feel uncomfortable burying your crystal directly in the ground, you can place it in a glass container and bury the container. It isn't necessary for the entire container to be covered in earth.

- If you are fortunate enough to live in the right area, burying your crystal in clean, fresh snow is a great way to cleanse and charge your crystal.

- Natural light is also a good way to go. Sunlight has a very cleansing effect on your crystals and can burn away any unwanted energy if you leave your crystals outside for an hour or two on a bright sunny day. There are some crystals like amethyst, aquamarine, fluorite, citrine, rose, and smoky quartz that lose some of their color when exposed to direct sunlight, but luckily moonlight works too. Moonlight has the same cleansing effect as sunlight, but it will take a little longer. The closer you are to a full moon, the stronger the effects. If you want to get an extremely thorough and potent cleansing and charging from the moon, you should put your crystals outside just after dusk and retrieve them shortly before dawn for twenty-eight consecutive days to expose the crystal to all the phases of a lunar cycle.

- Some crystals like clear quartz and carnelian have natural cleansing abilities, and you can use these to cleanse your other crystals. You can either place the crystal you want to cleanse on a larger cleansing crystal that will draw out the negative energy, or you could pack a circle of several small cleansing crystals around the crystal to be cleansed. These crystals may not need it as often as other types, but you shouldn't forget to cleanse your cleansing crystals every now and then too.

- Sage is a plant with many healing properties that can cleanse your crystal and restore its natural energy. To do this, set fire to some sage, it can be held in a bundle or loose in a fire-safe bowl, and move your crystal through the smoke of the sage. Thirty seconds of this should be enough, but if you feel the crystal needs a little more cleansing, add another thirty seconds. This process is called *smudging*, and should always be done outside or near a window.

- Probably one of the most simple and straightforward ways to cleanse a crystal is to leave it overnight in a bowl of brown rice. The brown rice will absorb all the negative and unwanted energy, and because of that, you shouldn't cook with it afterward. You can use the rice as compost, however.

- *Purple plates* or *positive energy plates* are devices sold at specialized stores and designed specifically to cleanse and charge your crystals. They are a great help but can be a little tricky to come by and tend to be slightly pricey. These plates aren't my first suggestion for beginners who are still just testing out the waters.

A good average to work by is cleansing your crystals about once a month, but you can never cleanse your crystals too often. A crystal in need of some cleansing will often feel slightly heavier, and you can feel its effects on you weakening. You'll also feel the presence of the negative energy within your crystals in severe cases. A cleansed crystal will feel lighter physically and in its energy. If you feel that a crystal is in need of cleansing, it doesn't matter how long ago you've cleansed it. You should cleanse it again. You should also cleanse your crystals before and after every meditation and healing session. If you're not carrying a crystal with you or have it placed in your home for a specific purpose, you should keep your crystals somewhere near windows and plants so they can constantly draw cleansing energy from nature and the sun and moon.

Charging Crystals

The same way people get tired at the end of the day and cellphone batteries die after a while, crystals will begin to lose their energy as they are used. There is only so much space for energy inside a crystal, and if it's used up completely, you will end up with a crystal that can barely do anything to heal or help you. This is a natural occurrence, and it is an easy solution to the problem: you simply need to charge the crystal with more energy. There various to charge crystals, and cleansing and charging can sometimes be done at the same time, using the same method. Here are some simple ways to charge your crystals:

- As with cleansing, you can expose your crystals to sunlight and moonlight for a few hours. Charging often takes longer than cleansing, and seven hours is a good general time frame, but how long you leave them exposed is up to you. It is important to make sure you don't expose the crystals to both sunlight and moonlight in the same charging session, as the two sources are quite different. If you're using sunlight to charge a crystal, exposing it to direct moonlight will change the energy in your crystal.

- Take your crystal to a place with a lot of nature, like a park or beach. Crystals can absorb positive, natural energy from the nature around them.

- Charge the crystal with some of your own energy. By keeping your crystal on you and focusing on sending your energy to the crystal, you can recharge the crystal using your own positive thoughts and energy.

- Again, just like with cleansing, water can be a great tool in recharging your crystals. Especially if you're using natural water or saltwater. The same goes for burying your grounding crystals in the earth.

- Fire is a great element for charging crystals. You can either do this by waving your crystal over a candle for a minute or so or by putting your crystals next to a fire for a short while. Be careful which crystals you use this method on and how long you leave them by the fire, as some types, such as amethyst, will change or lose their color if they are exposed to very high temperatures for too long.

- If you are willing to invest the money, purple plates and positive energy plates are designed to charge crystals as well as cleanse them.

- Smudging your crystals with sage will charge your crystals at the same rate that it will cleanse them.

- Crystals used for cleansing other crystals usually have a charging effect as well, and crystals that promote energy and physical activity can be very effective in giving energy to other crystals.

There is no set of rules for how frequently your crystals will need to be charged, and it is up to you to figure out what works for you. You should be able to feel if a crystal needs to be charged by the amount of energy you feel from it and how strongly it affects you when you're using it to heal, and you should charge your crystals whenever you feel they need it. In many cases, when you should charge a crystal depends on the crystal itself and how often you use them. Larger crystals tend to hold more energy than smaller ones, and some cuts and shapes are good for manifesting energy. These crystals don't need to be charged as often, but smaller crystals will lose their energy much faster. Crystals that are used frequently, such as those used for meditation, chakra aligning and healing sessions, will lose energy at a faster rate than those placed in rooms to gently radiate energy, and so should be charged more frequently. It's a good idea to charge these crystals before and after every time you use them. Crystal jewelry you wear constantly or crystals that you always keep in your purse or pocket will be the ones that need the most charging. Luckily it is also very easy to charge them with your own energy, which you can do while you go through your day, or quickly taking a detour to your nearest park or sitting in your garden with your crystals a while.

Crystals can be an important tool in improving your life and health, and cleaning, cleansing and charging them should become second nature to you if you want to use them to their best potential. By neglecting to care for your crystals properly, you rob them of their ability to heal and reduce them to nothing more than pretty decorations and interesting jewelry.

Chapter 6: Crystals from A-Z

The world is full of hundreds of different types of crystals, each with their own abilities, appearance, and traits. It might be a little difficult to learn everything there is to know about crystals, and memorizing the names, appearance, and abilities of even just a few crystals will take time. To help you get started so long and to provide a good guide for you, this crystal directory will focus mainly on crystals that are most commonly used and fairly easy to get your hands on. This directory will give you a clear description of every crystal, as well as their healing properties and where to find them.

Agate

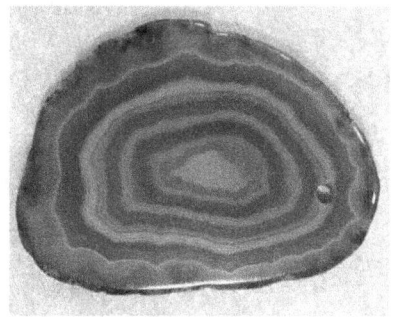

Agate is a crystal that comes in a wide variety of shapes and colors. It is a very common gemstone and easy to come by, but also very often faked. It is mainly mined in Africa, Brazil, Czech Republic, India, Morocco, and the United States.

Appearance: agate is often clear or milky white color, but it can also be gray, blue, pink, brown or green. It is often banded and can even be clear with fragments of colored crystal inside. It is a fairly soft crystal and often has a waxy appearance. It is often sold as tumbled stones or in polished thin slices, often with a ring of amethyst or quartz growing in the centre. Solid slices of agate are often just dyed glass with no healing properties, and agate often has its colors enhanced through dye.

Healing properties and uses: agate is a very stable stone that is often used for grounding. It can provide you with physical, intellectual, and emotional balance, as well as a balance of positive and negative energies. It is a calm and soothing stone that brings strength but works slowly. It encourages self-confidence and self-analysis. Agate enhances concentration, analytical abilities, and perception, making it easier to find practical solutions. This crystal also encourages truthful speaking and memories can be stimulated through agate with clear crystals within. This crystal helps grow love and courage and can help heal heartache and disappointment, making it good for healing emotional trauma. Agate leads to inner stability and spiritual growth by raising your consciousness of the world around you and encouraging you to experience life as much as possible. Agate can be used to remove negative energy and stabilize your aura. It can be used to heal the eyes, stomach, and uterus, as well as treat skin condition and strengthen blood vessels. It can also be used to cleanse the pancreas and can help stimulate the digestive system.

Amazonite

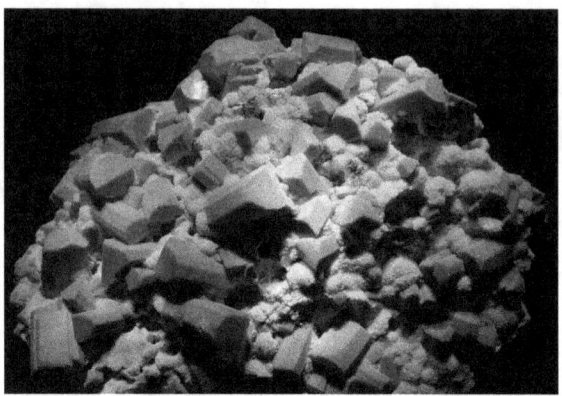

This crystal is very common and easy to come by. It is mined in Austria, Brazil, Canada, India, Mozambique, Namibia, Russia, and the United States.

Appearance: amazonite comes in shades of blue and green. It is an opalescent stone, meaning it reflects light in a way similar to opal, especially when it is cut and polished. It has a fairly uneven color and veins running through the crystal. It is most commonly sold as a raw or tumbled crystal.

Healing properties and uses: this crystal is considered a filtering stone, and can be used to protect you from electromagnetic pollution, cell phone emanations and microwaves, mostly by absorbing them. It is a soothing stone that increases intuition and balances many opposing traits in your personality, such as your masculine and feminine traits. It helps you see different angles and points of view in a situation and can soothe emotional trauma. It also helps remove negative emotional energy. It is strongly connected to the heart and throat chakras and helps develop universal love. Amazonite can heal blockages and negative energy in your nervous system, relieves and reduces muscle spasms, and balances metabolic deficiencies that may cause tooth decay and osteoporosis Amazonite also helps treat calcium problems if used in elixir form.

Amber

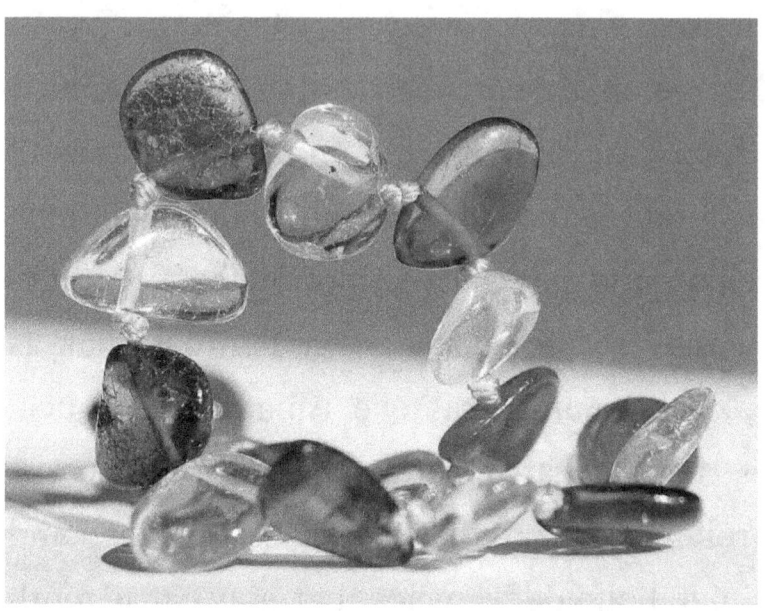

Amber may not technically be a crystal as it is petrified and fossilized tree sap, but it is still used as a crystal due to its healing properties. It is found mainly in Britain, Dominica, Germany, Italy, Myanmar, Poland, Romania and Russia, and is easily obtained in most parts of the world.

Appearance: amber is a transparent, translucent or opaque resin in a yellow or golden brown color. It is often polished and shaped, and there might be insects or bits of plants visible inside the amber.

Healing properties and uses: amber is strongly connected to the earth and nature, making it good for grounding energy. It is also a strong cleanser and healer, as it removes negative energy and encourages tissue revitalization. It is also good for healing and cleansing your chakras in general, as well as your aura. It transforms negative energy into positive energy that encourages the body to heal itself. It brings stability and motivation and encourages a positive mentality. This means it can be a good way to help prevent depression and suicidal tendencies. It also increases creativity and promotes self-expression. Amber also brings spiritual wisdom, patience, mental balance, and peacefulness. It aids the memory, helps develop trust in others and can improve your decision-making abilities. Amber can be used to give the body vitality and improve its ability to remove diseases. It absorbs pain and lessens stress, making it easier for the body to heal. Amber is good for treating the throat, stomach, liver, spleen, bladder, gallbladder, and kidneys. It can also help ease and reduce joint problems, and can be used to strengthen your mucus membranes. Amber is a great antibiotic when it comes to healing wounds and using it in elixir form.

Amethyst

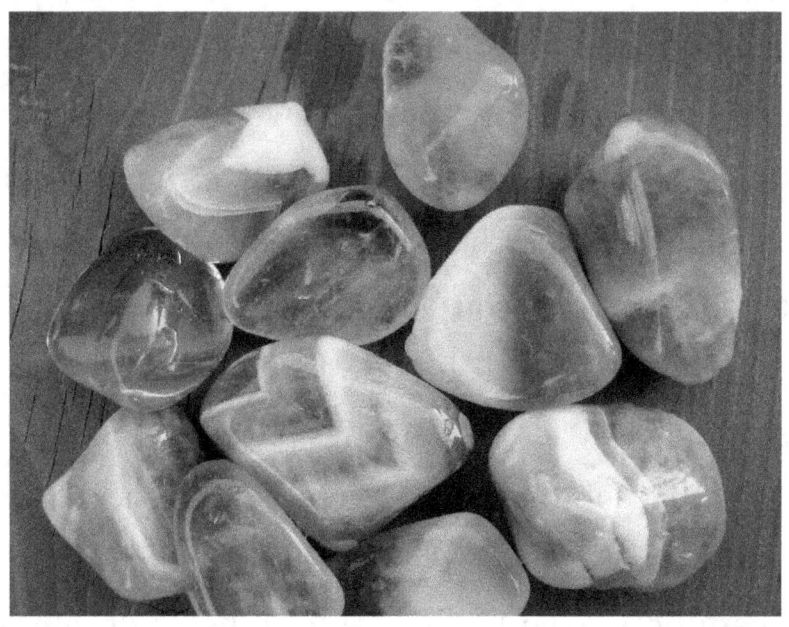

This is one of the most common crystals in the world, and you will be hard-pressed to find any type of crystal shop that doesn't have amethyst in stock. It is mainly mined in Brazil, Britain, Canada, East Africa, India, Mexico, Siberia, Sri-Lanka, Russia and the United States.

Appearance: this crystal comes in various shades of purple and violet and can vary from very translucent to opaque. It is found in all sizes and most often sold as crystal clusters, single crystal points, or inside geodes, but tumbled or shaped amethyst is not unusual.

Healing properties and uses: amethyst is a very spiritual stone that strengthens the third eye chakra, raises spiritual awareness and can protect you from negative psychic energy. It also enhances your own psychic abilities and can produce intuitive dreams and out-of-body experiences. It is a strong cleanser and healer and can be used as a powerful aid in meditation. It also clears the energy in the air around you, reduces certain types of stress, and acts as a natural tranquilizer. Amethyst has a long history of being worn to prevent hangovers and drunkenness and can be used to help prevent addictions. Amethyst can help you feel more focused and in control, and can both calm and stimulate the mind as is needed. It brings common sense and insight into the decision-making process, heals insomnia if it is caused by your mind being overactive, and protects against nightmares. Amethyst can also improve memory and motivation, making it a good stone to keep with you when preparing for and going through tests and exams. It balances your emotions and reduces negative emotions such as anger and anxiety. This crystal also alleviates grief and sadness, and it can be good for helping its wearer come to terms with loss. Although it should be avoided by those suffering from schizophrenia and paranoia, amethyst can help stabilize and better manage many other psychiatric conditions. Amethyst can be used to boost hormone production and the activity of your metabolism. It cleanses your organs and blood and strengthens the immune system. It reduces bruising and can be used to remove stress and reduce emotional, psychological and physical pain. If one reaches the end of their life, amethyst can be used to help the journey into the next life.

Variances and notes: amethyst reacts to high temperatures and changes its color to orange if exposed to intense heat too long. There are also some specific types of amethyst that have additional abilities.

Apatite

Apatite is a crystal that is available in a variety of colors and is found in Mexico, Norway, Russia, and the United States. While it is readily available in blue, it is rare to find a yellow apatite.

Appearance: this crystal is commonly opaque, but can be transparent on occasion. It has a very glassy surface and is found in a variety of sizes. It has a very hexagonal shape, and as such is usually sold raw or as a tumbled stone. Its colors are blue, brown, red-brown, gray, green, violet, white and yellow.

Healing properties and uses: this crystal is good for helping you find inspiration in the world around you, as well as to inspire you to do something new or different. It is a good stone to use in a crystal grid as it has strong manifestation abilities. It further helps deepen your meditation, strengthen spiritual attunement and develop and grow psychic abilities. It is a good crystal to use with the root chakra and encourages guiltless passion and removes frustration. This is also good for use with children who suffer from autism and hyperactivity. Apatite also improves communication. It helps soothe deep sadness, anger, and apathy, stimulates intellect and creativity, helps counter emotional exhaustion, and lessens irritability. It is good for building new cells in the body, overcoming hypertension, and healing the organs. This crystal also strengthens bones and teeth, aids calcium absorption, and is good for healing arthritis, rickets, and joint problems. Apatite is a great crystal to help you burn fat, as it encourages healthy eating, suppresses hunger, and speeds up your metabolism.

Apophyllite

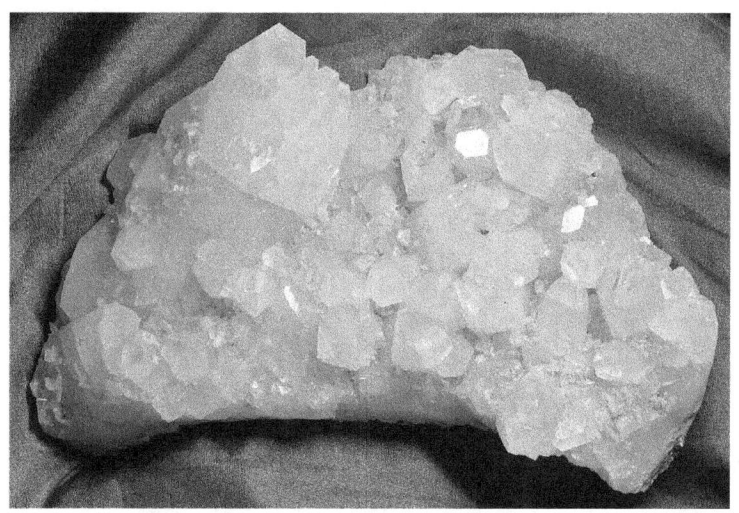

Apophyllite is readily available and found in Australia, Brazil, Britain, the Czech Republic, India, and Italy.

Appearance: apophyllite can range from transparent to opaque, but translucent apophyllite is a little bit rarer. Transparent crystals are often colorless, but apophyllite can be green, peach, white, or have a yellowish tinge. It tends to have a cube or pyramid shape and grows fairly small crystals. It grows abundantly, however, and large apophyllite clusters are quite common.

Healing properties and uses: this crystal acts well as a conductor and is strongly connected to the water element. It transmits vibrations very well and can amplify the energies within a room, making it great for enhancing the abilities of other crystals. It can help ground you to your physical body during deep meditation or out-of-body experiences and strengthens clear sight and intuition. Apophyllite encourages you to take a good look at your inner thoughts and emotions and helps fix the flaws and imbalances you find.it encourages truth, both to yourself and the world around you. It is a very calming stone that is good for stress relief and removing mental blocks. It puts the mind in tune with the spirit and encourages compassion and love when making decisions, and reduces desire.. This crystal helps reduce anxiety, overcome fear, and makes you more tolerant to uncertainty. This crystal is good for other types of energy-based healing, such as reiki healing, as it creates deep relaxation and enhances the transmission of energy. Apophyllite is good for the skin and sinuses, helps neutralize allergies, and can be held to the chest to stop asthma attacks. It is good for healing the spirit, and can greatly rejuvenate the eyes by placing a small apophyllite stone on each eyelid for a short while.

Aquamarine

Aquamarine is a well-known stone that is readily available and found in Afghanistan, Brazil, India, Ireland, Mexico, Pakistan, Russia, the United States, and Zimbabwe.

Appearance: this is another crystal that ranges from transparent to opaque. It has a blue-green color and is usually sold as a tumbled or faceted rough stone.

Healing capabilities and uses: aquamarine is a stone that is good for quieting the mind, providing quiet courage, and relieving stress. It also helps protect against pollutants. This stone has a history of gaining favor from light spirits and being worn as a talisman by sailors to protect them against drowning. Aquamarine is a good stone for those who are sensitive and is used as support by those overwhelmed. It can help you become less judgmental and more tolerant. It further encourages people to take responsibility for themselves. Aquamarine is ideal for removing unnecessary rogue thoughts, sharpens your mind and helps clear up any confusion. It encourages communication, self-expression, and closure. This stone is good for healing the throat chakra and strengthens clairvoyance. It is also a good stone to use during meditation. Aquamarine is a good crystal to use as a general immune booster, but it is especially good for healing throat problems. It helps strengthen the eyes, stomach, and teeth, and it's good for treating basic immune problems like hay fever.

Aragonite

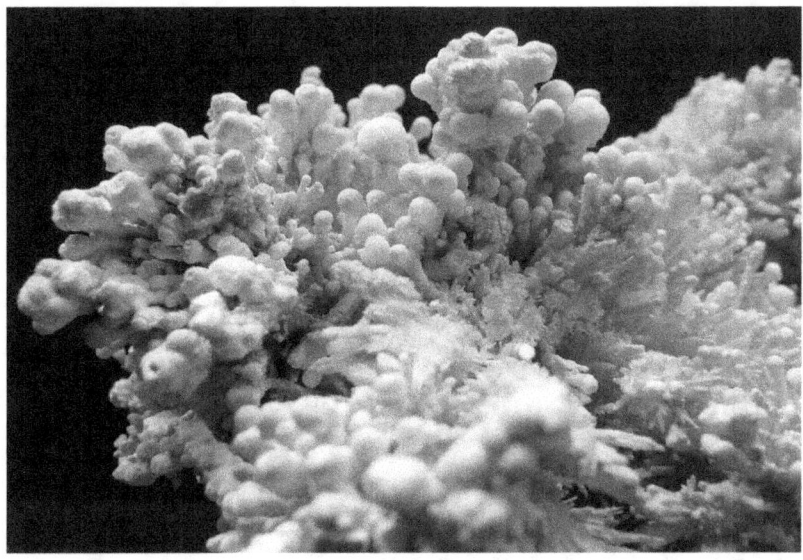

This crystal is mainly mined in Britain, Namibia, and Spain, but is easy to et your hands on all over the world.

Appearance: this crystal has mostly earthy colors like brown, gold and yellow, but can also be found in blue, green and white. It is either a transparent or translucent stone. It tends to be on the small side and has various different shapes, but usually has distinct protrusions. The most common shapes are a sputnik, fan and coral form.

Healing properties and uses: aragonite is a strong grounding stone and healer. It connects you to the earth, grounds your physical energy and can help relieve stress. It is also a very good stone for your root chakra. Aragonite can help develop tolerance, patience, flexibility of the mind and can improve concentration. It makes you feel secure and comfortable with yourself and provides emotional support in difficult times. Aragonite is good for preventing muscle spasms and twitching, helps warm cold extremities, strengthens bones and encourages the absorption of calcium, and helps lessen pain. It is a great tool for treating chills and Raynaud's Disease.

Beryl

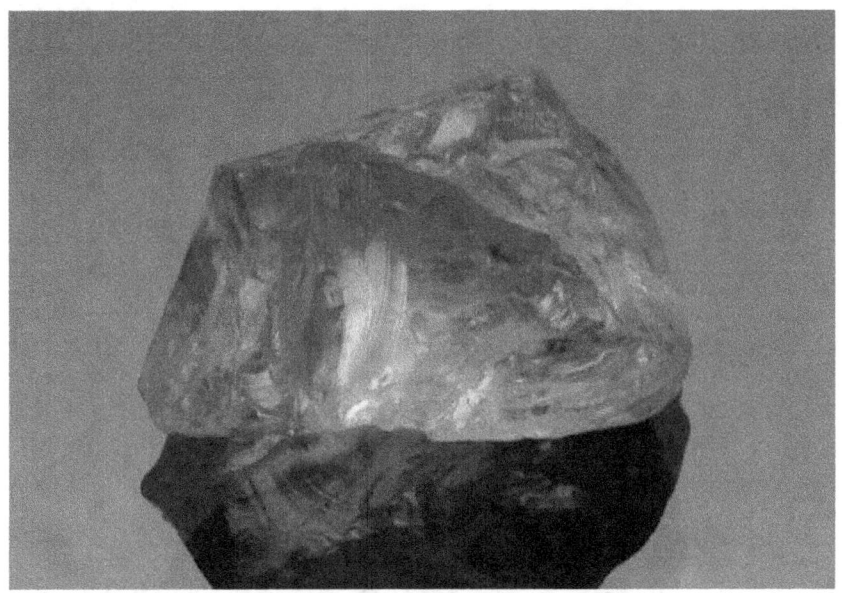

Beryl is a versatile stone that is found in Australia, Brazil, the Czech Republic, France, Norway, Russia, and the United States. It is sold in most forms and fairly easy to come by, but it can get expensive.

Appearance: beryl may be transparent or translucent. Its colors are blue, gold, green, pink, white and yellow. Although it is often cut into shapes or tumbled, it has a natural prism shape, but may also be more of a pyramid shape. It can vary from very large to very small.

Healing properties and uses: out of the stress-relieving stones, beryl is by far the strongest and is extremely good for helping you get rid of extra baggage that you don't need. This stone is often used for crystal balls, works very well with your solar plexus and crown chakras, and can help you bring out your full potential. Beryl can calm the mind by reducing anxiety, negativity, distraction, and overstimulation. It can help reawaken love that has begun to fade. This crystal can be used to strengthen your circulatory system and help you resist pollution and other toxins. It can be used to treat problems with the throat, heart, spine, liver, and stomach and is great for dealing with concussions. Beryl can further be used as a light sedative.

Bloodstone

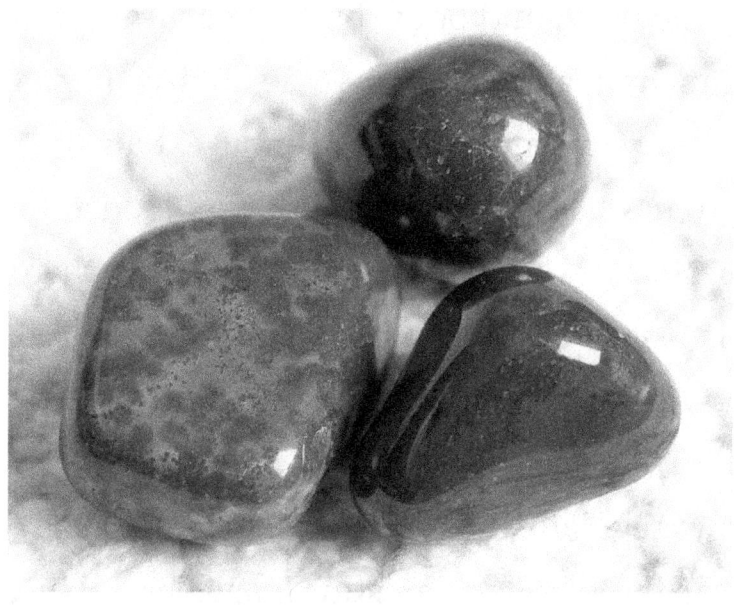

A powerful healing stone, bloodstone is readily available and originates from Australia, Brazil, China, the Czech Republic, India, and Russia.

Appearance: bloodstone is a red-green stone that consists mainly of green quartz with veins and flecks of yellow or red jasper. It is usually found in a medium size and is most often sold as a tumbled stone.

Healing properties and uses: this stone is marvelous when it comes to cleansing the blood, making it a very strong healer. This stone can help strengthen your intuition and creativity. It is good for revitalizing the mind and body, building courage and increasing mental and emotional flexibility. It can help you calm your mind, fight mental exhaustion, and adjust to new and unusual situations. Bloodstone is a good protector and helps ground you to the here and now. It also reduces negative emotions such as aggression, impatience, and irritability. Bloodstone can be used to clear infections, stimulate your metabolism, regulate blood flow, and act as a detoxifier for the bladder, intestines, spleen, kidney, and liver. This is also a great stone to use as an aid in cases like leukemia. Since ancient times, this crystal has been believed to be a magical tool full of mystical powers, such as controlling the weather, predicting the future and relaying it through sound, and banishing evil. The ancient Egyptians also used this stone to decrease the size of tumors.

Carnelian

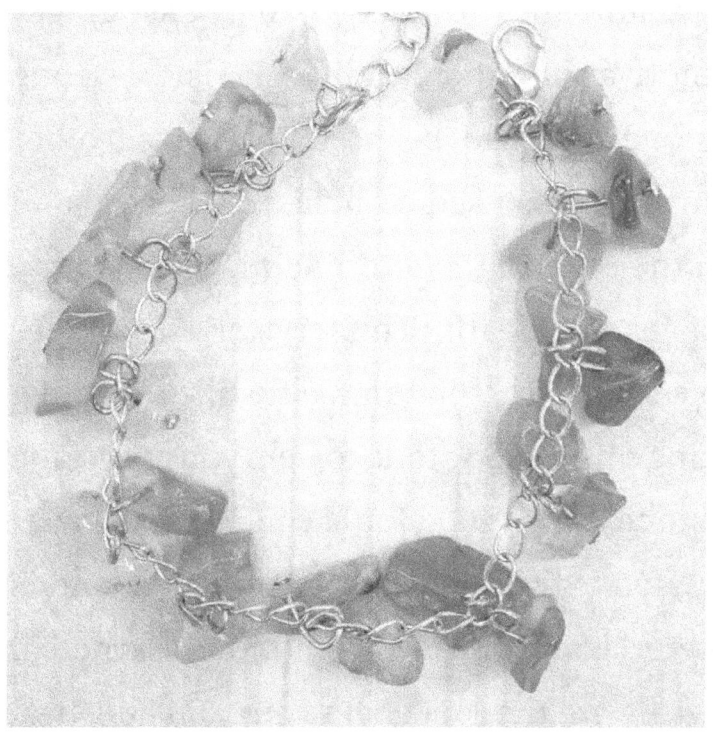

This is a very common crystal, making it easy to get your hands on. It is found in Britain, the Czech Republic, Iceland, India, Peru, Romania, and Slovakia.

Appearance: this stone is a relatively small, translucent crystal that is often water-worn. It is commonly sold as tumbled stone, and its natural colors are brown, orange, pink and red.

Healing properties and uses: carnelian is a stone with a large amount of energy that encourages creativity, motivation and vitality. It is a strong grounding stone that can be used to cleanse other crystals. Many cultures used carnelian as a guide and protector on the road to the afterlife due to its ability to remove a fear of death. This crystal encourages positive choices and trust in yourself while lessening apathy, making this a good stone to help you overcome abuse. This stone is also good for use in meditation, as it can help lessen extra, unnecessary thoughts, and is a good protector against negative emotions. Carnelian can be used well with the root chakra and can help heal depression, lower back problems, arthritis, and rheumatism. It helps the body absorb minerals and vitamins, making it good for healing ligaments and weak or injured bones. This crystal is very good for fighting impotence in men and improving fertility in women. It can aide in the stanching of bleeding and regulating the fluids within your body.

Citrine

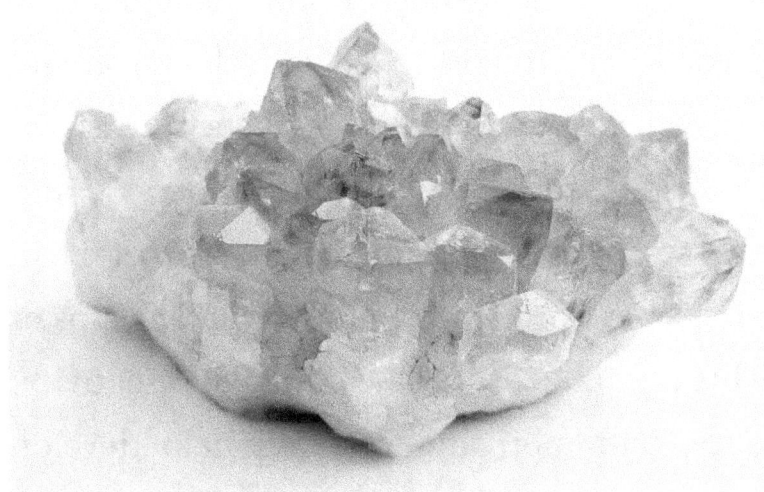

Citrine is a fairly rare crystal found in Brazil, Britain, France, Madagaskar, Russia, and the United States.

Appearance: citrine is a transparent or translucent crystal that has a gray-brown, yellow-brown or yellow color and grows in all sizes. It commonly forms in clusters or inside geodes, but it's often also sold as single citrine points.

Healing properties and uses: citrine is incredibly similar to amethyst in its healing abilities and the way it is used. Citrine is one of the few crystals that never needs to be cleansed, and is strongly connected to the sun and earth. It is also good for absorbing, grounding and transforming negative energy, making it great for cleansing your aura. It works well with the naval and solar plexus chakras and helps activate the crown chakra. Citrine radiates positive energy and encourages strong feelings of joy within a space. It can also help lessen discord among families and groups of friends. This crystal boosts self-confidence, creativity, individuality, and motivation. It can help develop optimism and a resistance to negative feelings and actions directed at you. This crystal improves concentration and expression of your thoughts and feelings. It is a very spiritual stone that helps gain wisdom and opens the higher mind. It balances you emotionally and removes negative emotions such as fear and anger. Citrine can give new energy to both the body and the mind, and it does great work in reversing the effects of degenerative diseases. It is good for healing bladder and kidney infections, helping blood circulation and digestion, and dealing with eye problems. This crystal is also good for the pancreas and spleen and can cleanse the blood. Citrine can do wonders to remove cellulite and can be taken as an elixir to balance the hormones and treat problems with menstruation and the symptoms of menopause.

Fluorite

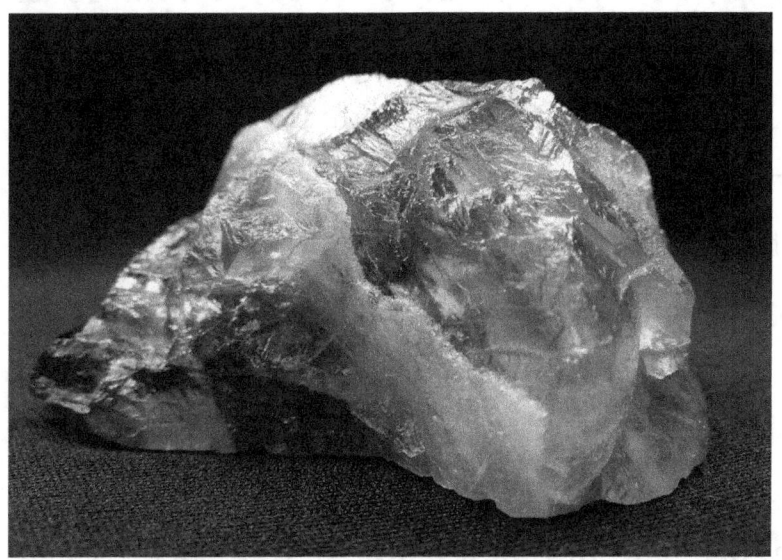

This crystal is very common and found in Australia, Brazil, Britain, China, Germany, Mexico, Norway, Peru, and the United States.

Appearance: fluorite is a transparent crystal that grows into all sizes and usually has a cube or octahedron type shape. Its colors are blue, brown, clear, green, purple, and yellow.

Healing properties and uses: this is a very protective crystals, especially against psychic energies. It is very good with cleansing and stabilising your aura and can relieve stress. Fluorite is very effective at drawing negative energy out of the body. It improves your intuition and can help bring organization into your life. It is a very spiritual stone useful in speeding up spiritual awakening. This crystal also improves your self-confidence and coordination, both mentally and physically. Fluorite can help you concentrate, absorb and process information and improve your ability to think quickly on your feet, making this crystal a good learning and studying aide. This crystal can stabilize you and help you stay impartial. It also helps you find balance physically and in relationships. Fluorite is often used to treat infections, viruses, wounds, and ulcers. It is very beneficial towards the skin, cells, teeth, and bones. This crystal is a good pain reliever and can be used to soothe arthritis, spine problems, and rheumatism. Fluorite can further help remove wrinkles and skin blemishes and increase your libido.

Hematite

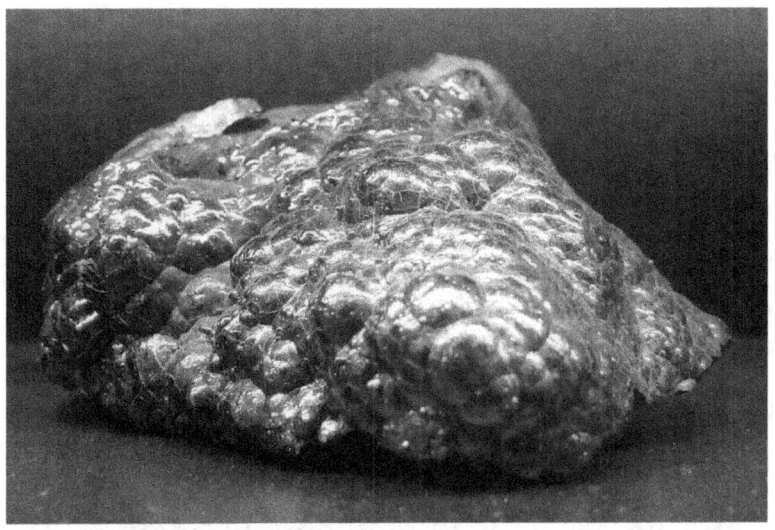

Hematite is a very common crystal found in Brazil, Britain, Canada, Italy, Sweden, and Switzerland.

Appearance: this crystal has an almost brain-like texture in appearance when it is raw, but is very reflective when polished. It is a very heavy stone that comes in all sizes and has a red or silver color.

Healing properties and uses: hematite is a very strong protector and grounding stone that can be used to find harmony between the mind, body, and spirit. It has also been strongly connected to the yang side of the yin yang concept. It is especially effective in warding off all negative energy. It provides emotional support, boosts your self-confidence and willpower, and makes you more reliable. Hematite is a very good stone to help you conquer addictions such as smoking and overeating. It can help you accept your failures and mistakes and learn from them. It helps you enhance your concentration and memory, and encourages original thinking. It can be used to lower fever and draw unwanted heat out of the body, and regulate and increase your blood supply, making it a good healing stone for cases such as anemia. It can help support tissue regeneration, treat circulatory problems, and help treat insomnia, muscle cramping, insomnia, bone fractures and problems with the alignment of your spine.

Jade

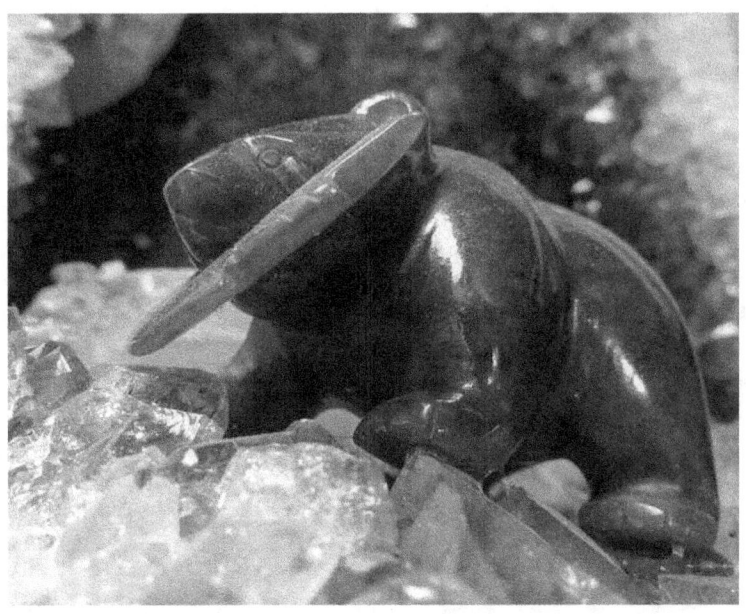

This stone is considered very sacred in some cultures and is found in China, Italy, the Middle East, Myanmar, Russia, and the United States. It is divided into two sub-categories called *nephrite* and *jadeite*, of which Nephrite is the more easily obtainable. Jade is generally available all over the world, but there are some colors that are quite rare.

Appearance: jade is found in blue, blue-green, brown, cream, green, lavender, orange, red and white. Jadeite is a more translucent crystal, while nephrite has a creamy appearance. It is available in all sizes, and the surface has a slightly soap-like texture to the touch.

Healing properties and uses: jade is strongly associated with purity, serenity, tranquility, and wisdom. It is connected to the heart chakra, meaning it encourages love, especially the nurturing kind. Jade is a very stabilizing stone that gets rid of negative thoughts and energy, promotes swift action and encourages you to be more self-sufficient. It is a calming stone that encourages you to be yourself and releases negative emotions such as irritation and impatience. Jade is very good for the kidneys and spleen and helps improve fertility. It can be of assistance during childbirth and is often used to heal stitched wounds. Jade helps rebuild your cells and skeleton and balance the fluids in your body. Jade has long been considered very lucky and is believed to attract friendship.

Jasper

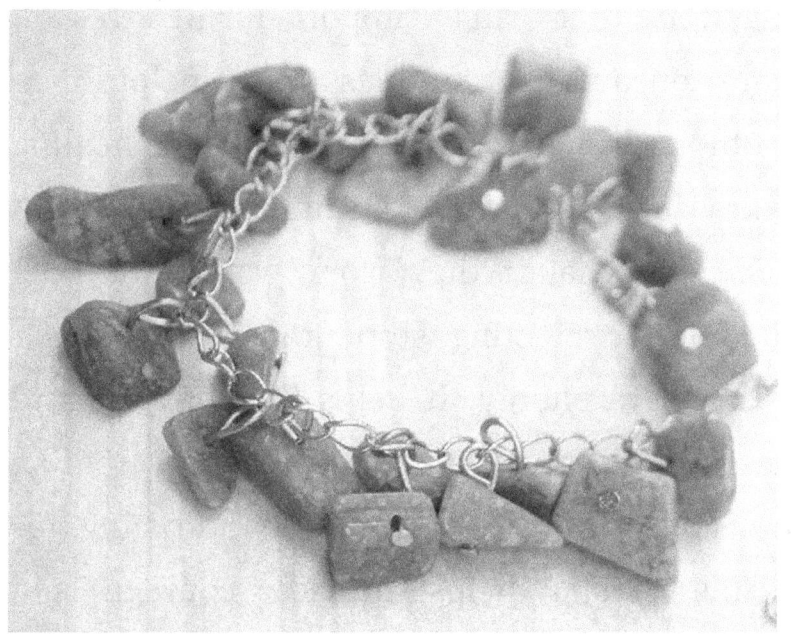

This is another of the most common gems out there and can be found worldwide. It can also be found lying openly on the ground here and there in naturally rocky areas.

Appearance: this is an opaque stone that usually has a pattern of some sort and is often found as a water-worn stone. It is usually sold as a small tumbled stone. Its colors are blue, brown, green, purple, red and yellow, with red and brown being the most common.

Healing properties and uses: this is an extremely nurturing stone that brings support during stressful times and encourages kindness and helpfulness towards others. Jasper is good for aligning and healing your chakras in general, while the different colors each have a specific chakra they work well with. It is grounding and protecting stone that absorbs and cleanses negative energy. It helps find balance and helps clear pollution. It is especially good at treating radiation. Jasper is often used when dowsing for water. This crystal helps provide courage and determination and encourages you to be honest with yourself. This crystal helps strengthen the imagination and quick thinking abilities. Jasper is beneficial to the sexual organs, as well as organs relating to the digestive and circulatory systems, and it helps manage and balance the minerals within your body.

Jet

This stone is fairly easy to come by. It can be found all over the world, but it is especially abundant in the United States.

Appearance: this is a black stone that has an appearance similar to coal, especially in its raw form. It is commonly sold as a small, polished stone. Jet is formed when wood is fossilized.

Healing properties and uses: jet is a strong barrier stone that can ward off negative energy and fear, especially if that fear is unreasonable. This stone can help you gain spiritual enlightenment and open yourself to psychic experiences. This stone needs special attention when it comes to cleansing, especially if it is used for healing purposes. Jet can be used to help you take better control of your life and fight against depression. It can bring balance and stability and is especially effective in cleansing the root chakra. It is good for managing epilepsy, migraines, colds, swelling, and stomach pain, and it has a tradition of being used to lessen the intensity of menstrual cramps.

Kyanite

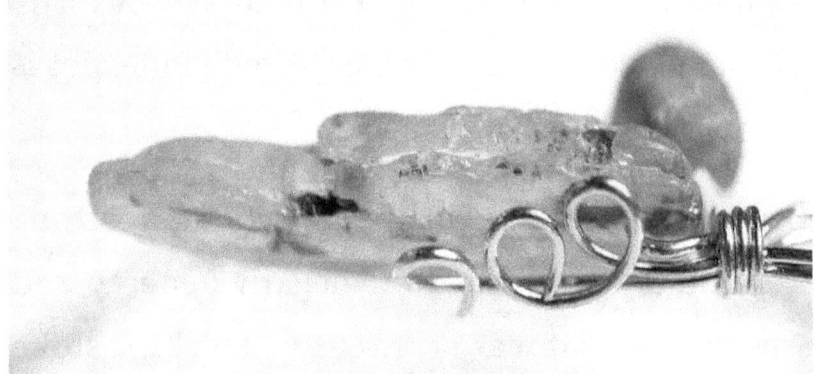

This crystal is only found in Brazil, but it's fairly easy to come by all over the world.

Appearance: this is a crystal that often consists of small blades of stone grown together. It can either be opaque or transparent and is often pearlized. It can be found in all sizes and its colors are black, blue-white, gray, green, pink and yellow.

Healing properties and uses: kyanite has a strong ability to amplify energies and improving intuition and psychic abilities. It brings tranquility and is a good stone to use for meditation. This crystal encourages compassion and spiritual maturity and is another stone that can help ease the journey into death.

Kyanite is good for working with the throat chakra and encourages truth and communication, while also helping overcome fear and other blockages. It can help remove anger, frustration, confusion, and stress. It strengthens your linear and logical thinking capabilities and helps you better understand your place in the world. It is a stone that does not hold any negative energy and thus doesn't need to be cleansed. Kyanite is used to treat fevers, problems with the brain, adrenal glands, the urogenital system, the thyroid, and muscle disorders. This stone can be used to treat infections and lower blood pressure, and it acts as a natural pain reliever. It can help improve your body's motor skills and get rid of extra weight, as well as support the cerebellum.

Labradorite

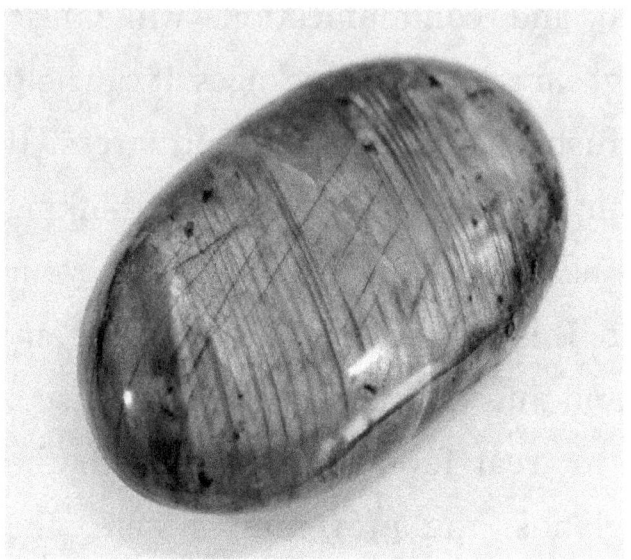

Labradorite is a stone found in Canada, Finland, Greenland, Italy, Russia, and Scandinavia, and it's readily available.

Appearance: labradorite can either be varying shades of grey and black with traces of blue, or yellow. Dark labradorite is an opaque stone that usually has a reflective surface when polished, and has gold or blue iridescent streaks. It is available in all sizes. Yellow labradorite is a transparent stone that tends to be small and is most commonly sold as a tumbled stone.

Healing properties and uses: if labradorite is iridescent, it is a very protective stone that can ward off unwanted energy and keep you from losing your own energy through leakages. It helps strengthen psychic gifts and intuition, get rid of insecurity and fear, and can calm your mind if it is overactive. It can also help bring up past memories that are usually suppressed. Labradorite can give your perseverance and inner strength a boost, especially in times of change. It is used to lessen stress and menstrual tension, treat disorders in the brain and eyes and lower blood pressure. It is a good healer for rheumatism, colds, and gout.

Lapis Lazuli

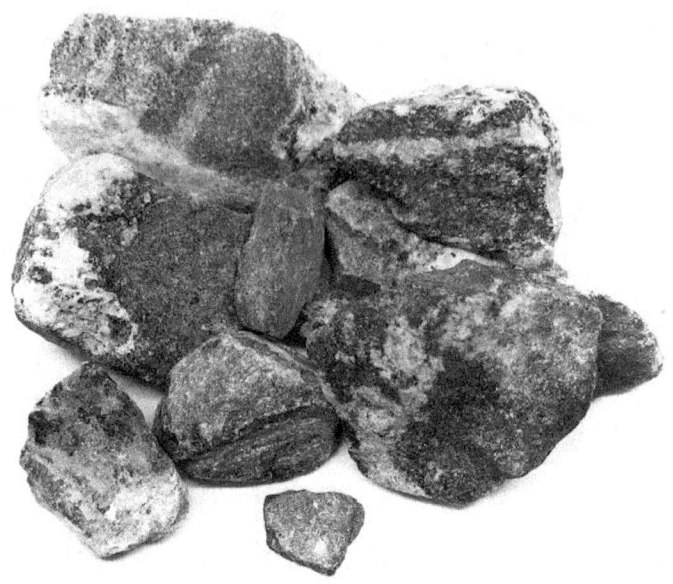

This is a stone often associated with royalty and magic in history and fantasy works. It is found in Afghanistan, Chile, Egypt, Italy, the Middle East, Russia, and the United States. Although it is easy to come by lapis lazuli in stores, it does tend to be expensive. It is often also simply called *lapis*.

Appearance: lapis is a very dense stone with deep blue color and golden veins and flecks. It comes in all sizes, and although it is usually polished and shaped, it is sometimes also sold as a tumbled stone. Many people describe lapis lazuli as resembling the night sky.

Healing properties and uses: this stone is good for using with the throat and third eye chakras, and can do much to enhance psychic abilities. It can help strengthen your personal spiritual power and can protect you from negative psychic energy. If you feel an intense lack of purpose or depression, lapis can be a good stone to help you fight against these problems. It can remove stress, encourage truth and self-expression, and helps you take charge of your life. Lapis lazuli helps you reach a better understanding of yourself and work through repressed anger. It brings compassion, honesty and a strong sense of justice and fairness, which is part of why the Egyptians often used this in the jewelry of pharaohs. It can help you find clarity and stay objective when necessary but also brings creativity. This stone helps strengthen loving relationships and friendships and can be used to settle and lessen conflict. It can help you better express your emotions and face difficult truths, but also helps remove emotional bondage. Lapis lazuli is used as a strong pain reliever, especially against migraines, as well as to lower blood pressure. It is good for healing most throat maladies, strengthening your immune system and cleansing bone marrow and organs. It's good for your nervous and respiratory systems, can purify blood, and helps fight vertigo and insomnia. In many cultures throughout history, lapis lazuli was used to remove curses and contain guardian spirits.

Lepidolite

This stone is easy to get your hands on and is found in Brazil, the Czech Republic, the Dominican Republic, Madagascar, and the United States.

Appearance: it is either pink or purple, and can have a grainy texture or have a slightly shiny surface. It grows in thin plate-like layers and can be found in all sizes. Its properties are extended to a great extent when lepidolite has a mica form.

Healing properties and uses: a good place to keep this stone is near computers and televisions, as it can help remove electromagnetic pollution. It gets rid of all types of negativity and can help you overcome spiritual and emotional blockages. It is good for activating your heart, throat, third eye and crown chakras. It is an exceptional tool against stress and depression that can help you break away from addictions, obsessive thoughts, and mental and emotional dependence. It can help you become more independent, stay objective, make quick decisions and filter out unnecessary distractions. Lepidolite can be used to fight anorexia and insomnia, stabilize mood swings, and better manage bipolar disorders. It improves concentration and analytic thinking and enhances your intellect. It is a calming stone that can help bring emotional healing. Lepidolite is used to help strengthen your immune system and relieve allergies and epilepsy, treat Alzheimer's and lessen exhaustion. It is good for healing joint problems and removing toxins from connective tissue and skin. It can also be used as an elixir to manage menopause.

Malachite

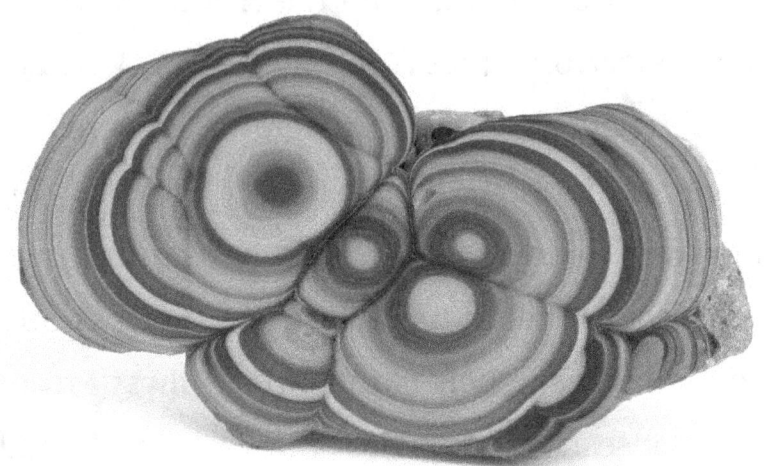

This stone is found in the Democratic Republic of the Congo, the Middle East, Romania, Russia, and Zambia, and it's easily obtained.

Appearance: this is a green crystal with layers of dark and light rings and rosettes. It can be found in all colors and is usually polished or tumbled.

Healing properties and uses: malachite is a powerful healer, but should be handled very carefully. It contains many toxic minerals that can be harmful even if just malachite dust is dangerous, so it should not be used as an elixir or in its raw form. Using this crystal under the supervision of a trained professional is best. Malachite can amplify positive and negative energy, but grounds spiritual energy. It is a protector stone that cleanses negative energy and pollution and protects against radiation. This stone is good for activating the chakras and can be placed on the third eye to activate psychic vision. It can also help open your heart to unconditional love. Malachite encourages change and a sense of adventure. It further helps you take responsibility for your actions, break away from unwanted ties, and express yourself better. It strengthens your insight and intuition and also your sense of empathy. This stone can help you better understand difficult ideas and concepts, and makes you more observant, and is good for treating mental disturbances and dyslexia. It further helps deep emotional healing and can help overcome old trauma and emotional hurt. One drawback of malachite is that it needs to be cleansed very often. Malachite is a very versatile stone and can be used for many types of healing, but it is especially effective against all types of cramps, asthma, epilepsy, growths, swollen joints, arthritis, tumors, vertigo and motion sickness. It can help make childbirth easier and is beneficial towards your immune system, optic nerves, pancreas, and spleen. Malachite can be worn around the waist to help manage diabetes and can lower blood pressure.

Moonstone

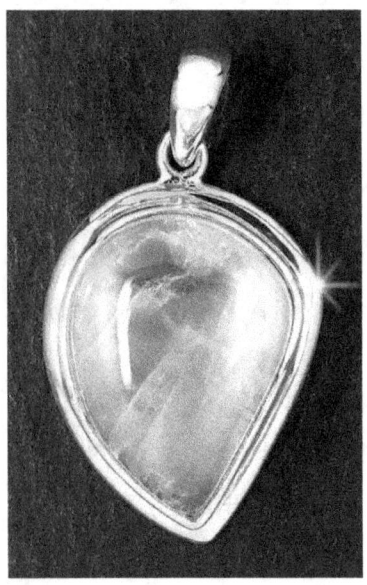

This well-known crystal is found in Australia, India, and Sri Lanka and is easy to come by.

Appearance: this stone is translucent with a milky appearance. It is found in all sizes and its colors are blue, cream, green, white, and yellow.

Healing properties and uses: this stone is strongly connected to the moon, and is named accordingly. Its strongest healing property is its ability to calm emotions. It is also strongly connected to and beneficial for your intuition, and is good for developing empathy. This stone can greatly improve psychic abilities and can encourage lucid dreaming. These effects are especially strong during a full moon. Moonlight is also the best way to cleanse and charge this crystal. This stone can help prevent overreactions and balances the masculine and feminine energies within your body. It is especially useful for men who want to get in touch with their feminine side and women who are overly aggressive. Moonstone can help open the mind, but also runs the risk of responding to wishful thinking with illusions. It can help you calm and soothe your emotions and find stability, as well as enhance your emotional intelligence. It also brings deep emotional healing. This crystal is very beneficial towards female reproductive organs and can be used to manage problems regarding menstruation. Moonstone helps treat hyperactive children and is very useful when someone is in a state of shock. It helps balance hormones and is a great healing tool to assist with all phases of pregnancy, from conception to childbirth. It is also great for managing PMS. Moonstone is good for removing toxins from the body and combating degenerative diseases regarding the skin, eyes, hair and certain organs such as the pancreas and liver. In elixir form, this stone can prevent sleepwalking and insomnia.

Obsidian

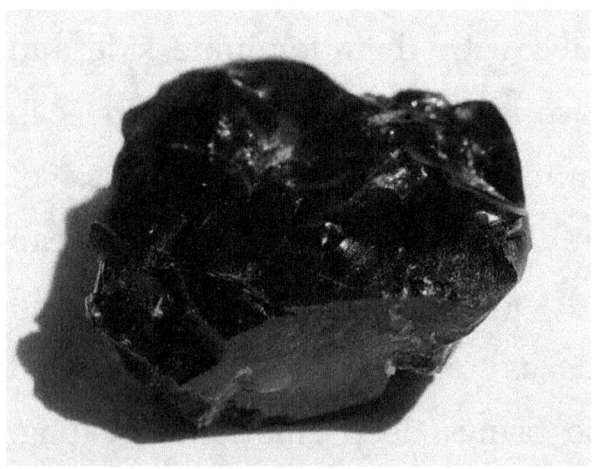

Obsidian is a stone that forms when lava cools too quickly to crystallize. It is found worldwide, but especially in Mexico. While some colors are fairly easy to come by, other, rarer colors are not. There are some colors like blue-green that are nothing more than shaped and treated glass.

Appearance: it is an opaque stone that has a very reflective, glass-like texture. It sold in all sizes in its raw form, but can sometimes be found as a tumbled stone. Its colors are black, blue, brown, green, red-black or silver. It can also have several colors on one stone, referred to as *rainbow*, or it can have a golden sheen.

Healing properties and uses: obsidian is a very powerful stone that works fast. It encourages truth and is good at bringing weaknesses, flaws and blockages into the light. This stone helps encourage you to grow as a person and supports you during this process. Because it can reveal unpleasant truths and negative emotions so strongly, it should be treated carefully and professional supervision is advised. Still, obsidian has the potential to bring about deep healing of the soul. It is a barrier stone that can ward off negativity of any kind, and is good for grounding and strengthening the root chakra. It can also protect you against negative psychic and spiritual energy. Many find obsidian to be an overwhelming stone, but many therapists find it to be a very useful tool. Obsidian can be a good stress reliever that has a calming effect and can help remove tension. It also helps you face your problems and find a permanent solution to them. Obsidian is good for removing confusion and binging clarity. This crystal needs to be cleansed very often due to the amount of negative energy it absorbs. It is used to remove blockages, tension and toxins from your body, is beneficial to the digestive system and blood circulation, and can lessen pain in cases of cramps, problematic joints, injuries, and arthritis. It can be effective at treating problems regarding hardened arteries and an enlarged prostate.

Onyx

This is a readily available stone that is found in Brazil, Italy, Mexico, Russia, South Africa, and the United States.

Appearance: it is a stone with rings and an often marble-like appearance. It is usually sold as a polished stone in all sizes. Its colors are black, blue, brown, gray, red, white, and yellow.

Healing properties and uses: onyx is a very supportive stone that gives strength during stressful, confusing and difficult times. It can help center your energy and can give you more vigor and stamina, as well as make you more steadfast. It helps you be more comfortable with the world around you and improves your self-confidence. It is very good for treating old injuries, trauma, and grief. It can help you get rid of fear and worry, and make better decisions, and helps improve your self-control. Obsidian helps strengthen your body's ability to heal naturally and is used to treat problems relating to the blood, bones, teeth, bone marrow and feet.

Opal

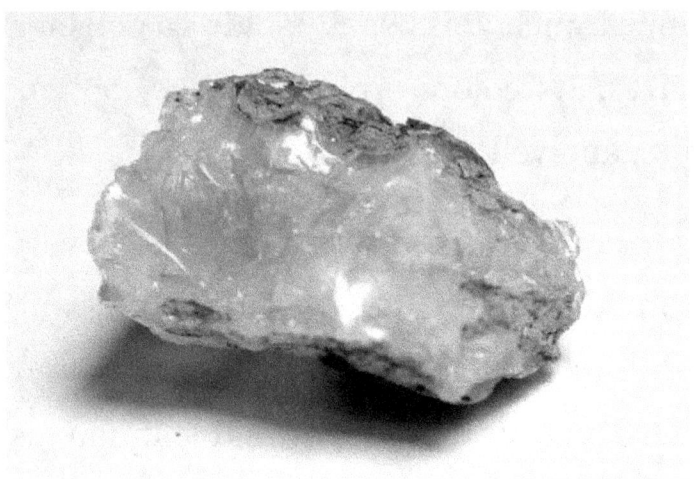

Opal is found in Australia, Britain, Canada, Honduras, Mexico, Peru, Slovakia, South America, and the United States. It is easy to come by, but it is expensive in gem form.

Appearance: this crystal has many variances. It can range from transparent to opaque and can be clear, milky, fiery, and/or iridescent. It often looks like glass, and is usually small and sold as a polished stone. It also has an incredibly beautiful way of reflecting light in different colors. Its colors are beige, black, blue, brown, clear, green, orange, pink, purple, white and yellow.

Healing properties and uses: this stone is excellent for inspiring creativity and originality, and can help you better express yourself. Opal is good for encouraging transformation within yourself and can help you bring more obscure and hidden traits of yourself to the surface. It can help you understand yourself and your full potential better, help you be more spontaneous, and strengthen your will to live fully. This crystal is long associated with love, desire, passion, and eroticism, and it can enhance these feelings, as well as other emotional states. It can help you let go of inhibitions, make it easier for you to approach others, and can stabilize your emotions, but it also has the ability to scatter your energy, and you should be able to keep yourself centered fully in difficult situations if you want to use opal in connection with your emotions. It is believed that opal can inspire loyalty and trust in a relationship if worn as a pendant, but it can also strengthen any fickle thoughts or tendencies that already exist. Opal is good for dealing with infections, problems with your eyes, fevers, and Parkinson's. It is good for cleansing your liver and blood, and can help ease childbirth, improver memory functions, and manage your insulin levels. Dark-colored opals are good for managing PMS.

Peridot

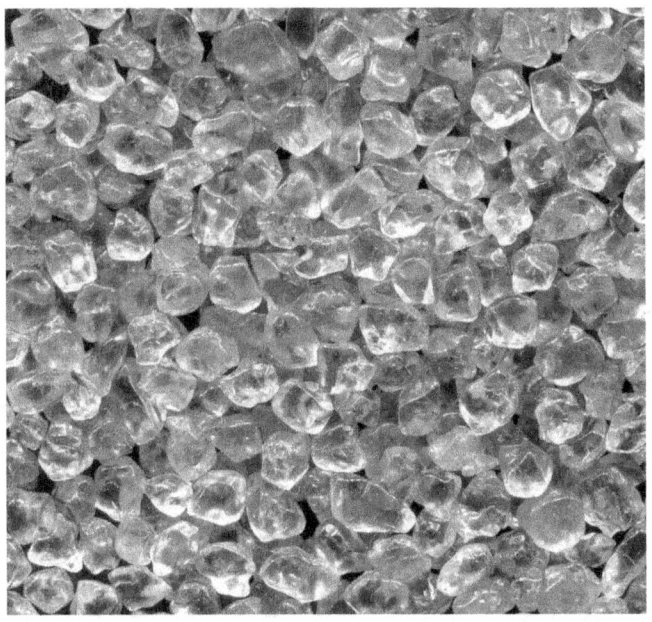

Peridot is easy to get your hands on, but high-quality crystals with few or no flaws are fairly rare. It is found in Brazil, the Canary Island, Egypt, Ireland, Russia, Sri Lanka, and the United States.

Appearance: it can have a brownish, honey, olive green, red, or yellow-green color. It appears as an opaque stone in its raw form, but becomes transparent when faceted or polished. It tends to be a fairly small crystal.

Healing properties and uses: peridot protects your aura and has very powerful cleansing properties. It is good at counteracting toxins and can help purify and activate the solar plexus and heart chakras. It can help remove negative elements of your life such as obsessions, heavy burdens, jealousy, anger, and guilt. It can help you let go of unnecessary attachments and helps you find clarity and wellness on a psychological level. It will help you overcome feelings of lethargy and make it easier for you to recognize and admit your own mistakes. Peridot can help you take more responsibility for your life and can be a great aid in difficult relationships. It is used to heal problems regarding damaged tissue, the heart, lungs, gallbladder, spleen, eyes, ulcers, and intestinal tract. It can be used to ease childbirth by placing it on the abdomen, which will ease much of the pain and strengthen the muscle contractions. It is good for treating hypochondria and balancing bipolar disorders. Peridot was used to ward off evil spirits in ancient times.

Pyrite

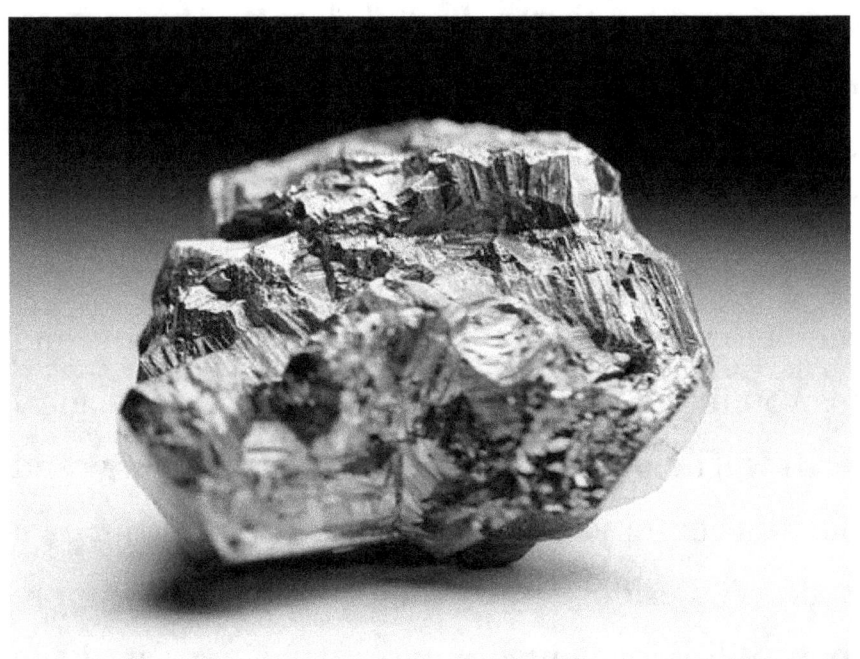

This crystal is also known as *iron pyrite* or, more commonly, *fool's gold*. It is commonly found in Britain, Chile, North America, and Peru, and it's readily available.

Appearance: Pyrite will have a brownish or gold color, and it tends to be a small to medium size. It often resembles gold in its raw form, but can also often have a cubic shape.

Healing properties and uses: pyrite is a protective stone that is especially effective against negative energy, and preventing energy leaking away from you. This stone contains a lot of positivity and can help conquer feeling inadequate and negative about yourself. It is good for gaining access to your unused abilities and potential and encourages diplomacy. It is good for raising your self-worth and removing frustration and anxiety from your life. It builds confidence and helps you find balance between your creative and analytic sides. Pyrite increases the flow of blood to your brain, increasing your mental activity and improving your memory. It is good for dealing with feelings of melancholy and despair, and it can give your body new energy. Pyrite works quickly and is good for your circulatory system. It is used to encourage cell formation and heals problems regarding damaged DNA and bones. It is very beneficial towards the digestive tract and respiratory system and the lungs. It can be used to treat asthma and bronchitis and counter the effects of toxins that have been ingested.

Quartz

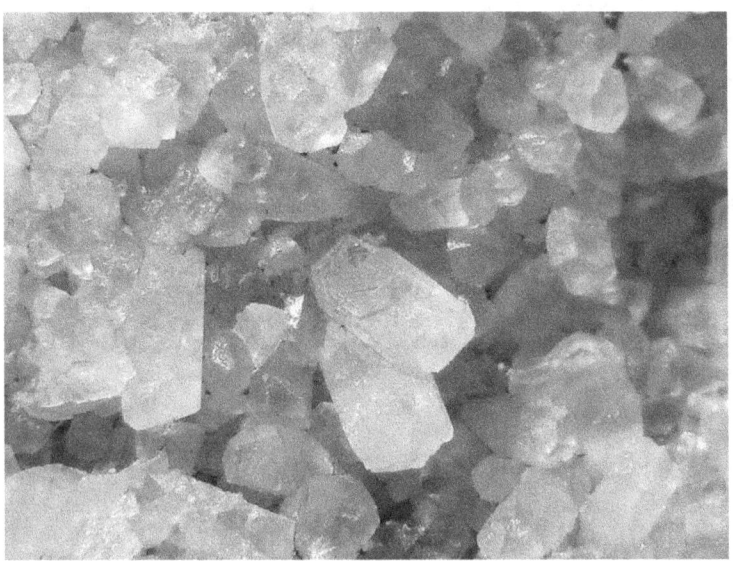

Quartz is a crystal group with various different types. Most of these types are exceptionally easy to come by and is found worldwide. It is another type of stone that can be easily found on the ground in rocky areas.

Appearance: your basic quartz is generally a clear stone, but there are color variants out there. This is a crystal that grows into any size and tends towards long crystal points. It is also often found in crystal clusters.

Healing properties and uses: this is the most powerful crystal when it comes to healing and amplifying the energy of other stones and people. It is good for unblocking the flow of energy and has the ability to absorb, regulate, store, and release energy. This crystal is good for protecting against radiation and getting rid of static electricity. It is also good for doing some deep soul cleansing work. Quartz can be used to remove distractions while meditation and strengthen psychic abilities. It helps give you access to locked memories. It is very easy to program this crystal. Quartz can be used to treat any ailment, but it is especially beneficial towards the immune system, and an excellent way to soothe burns, in many cases, acupuncture needles are coated with quartz to greatly strengthen their effects.

Rose Quartz

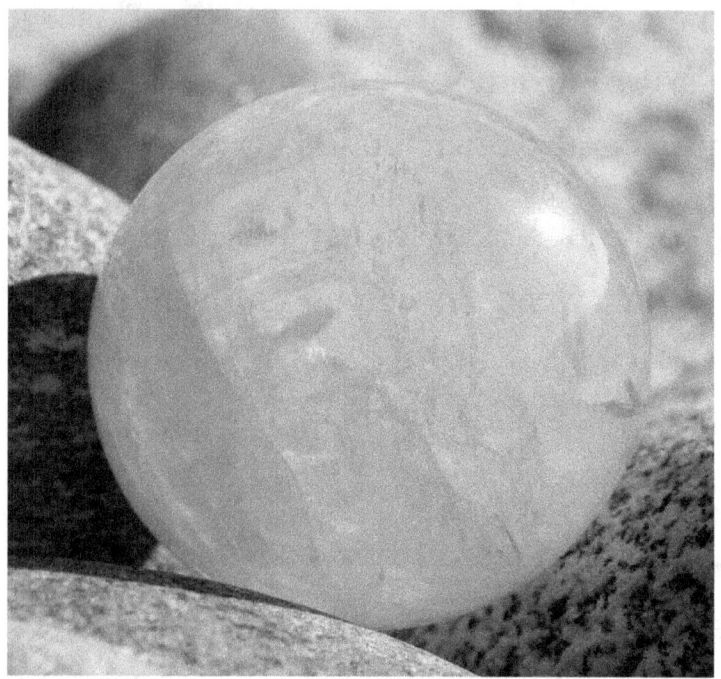

Although this crystal is a type of quartz, it is very different from your basic clear quartz and has its own set of healing properties, making it an individual crystal type. It is easy to come by and is found mainly in Brazil, India, Japan, Madagascar, and South Africa.

Appearance: it is usually a translucent stone, but can also occasionally be transparent. It has a pink color, can be found in all sizes, and is often sold as a tumbled stone.

Healing properties and uses: rose quartz is very deeply connected and encourages love for yourself and others. It is good to use during times of crisis or trauma, as it brings calmness and reassurance. It can be used to attract love and strengthen existing romantic relationships. Quartz can draw away different types of negative energy and can help develop empathy. It helps you deal with and accept change and promotes emotional healing on all possible levels. It helps you open yourself to the love and care of others and can help you overcome the grief of lost love. It can also help you forgive, accept and love yourself. Rose quartz is used to support the circulatory system and heart, treat Parkinson's, Alzheimer's, and dementia, and lessen feelings of vertigo. It is beneficial towards the lungs, kidneys, and skin, and it can be used to ease the pain from burns and blisters.

Smoky Quartz

This is another variant of quartz that can also be seen as its own crystal type. It is found worldwide and easy to come by, but it is often faked and treated to enhance the color, so be cautious when purchasing this type of crystal.

Appearance: the color of this translucent crystal ranges from brown to black, but can also be yellow. It can be found in all sizes and forms long crystal points, the tips of which tend to be darker than the rest of the crystal.

Healing properties and uses: smoky quartz is deeply connected to the earth and is considered the most powerful grounding stone. It brings stability, but can also be used during meditation. It is a good stone to help strengthen your resolve and get rid of stress. It is good for removing both negative energy and toxins and provides positive energy at the same time. It is good for fighting depression, fear, and suicidal tendencies, and brings calmness to your mind and body. It strengthens the root chakra and can increase your virility. It improves your concentration and communication abilities, encourages positive thinking and wards off nightmares. Smoky quartz is good for treating the negative effects of chemotherapy and other types of radiation-related problems. It can be used to relieve pain and treat ailments in the abdomen, legs, and hips. It is very beneficial toward the reproductive system, heart, and nerve and muscle tissue. It can help resolve back problems and is very effective against cramps and headaches. It also helps your body absorb necessary minerals.

Ruby

Because of its hardness and thus the difficulty of cutting and polishing, ruby is a very expensive gemstone. As a raw crystal, however, it is considerably cheaper, and not that difficult to come by. It is mined in Cambodia, India, Kenya, Madagascar, Mexico, Russia, and Sri Lanka.

Appearance: ruby is known for its bright red color. It is naturally an opaque crystal but becomes transparent when it is polished. Smaller pieces tend to form facets, while larger pieces have a more cloud-like shape.

Healing properties and uses: ruby provides energy and a healthy type of passion for life. It helps you set goals for yourself that reasonable and realistic, and gives you the motivation to see them through. It is strongly connected to the heart chakra but still has the ability to protect you from negative psychic energy. Ruby encourages leadership and helps you remove all negativity from life. Ruby is extremely beneficial to the mind, as it heightens your concentration and awareness. It also promotes positive thoughts and helps you become and stay confident. This stone brings enthusiasm and can improve potency, and can even be used to attract and increase sexual activity. Ruby can also be used to get rid of feelings of lethargy and physical exhaustion. It is a good detoxifier for the entire body, especially the blood, and can be used to help heal infectious diseases and fever. It can be of great help to the circulatory system and heart and is great for treating restricted blood flow. It also holds a great advantage for the spleen, adrenal glands, kidneys, and reproductive organs. Despite its ability to give energy and vigor, this stone can be a great tool to calm those who are hyperactive.

Selenite

This crystal is easily obtained and found in Austria, England, France, Germany, Greece, Mexico, Poland, Russia, and the United States.

Appearance: this stone is can be translucent and have fine ribbing, called satin spar, or rougher ribbing. It can also be more opaque and have a fishtail type shape. In the case of desert roses, the selenite forms a more petal-like shape. Its colors are brown, blue, green, orange, or pure white.

Healing properties and uses: translucent selenite is especially strong with the crown chakra if it's translucent. All selenite can bring calm and peace into your life and strengthen certain psychic abilities such as telepathy. This crystal is good for using in protective type crystal grids and meditation. It is good for improving your insight and judgment, getting rid of confusion, and bringing stability to or removing erratic emotions. It is used to help align the spinal cord and can prevent epileptic seizures. It can counteract the effects of mercury poisoning and improve your flexibility. This crystal is good for lending support and healing energy to mothers who are breastfeeding and trying to raise their children in a nurturing environment.

Sodalite

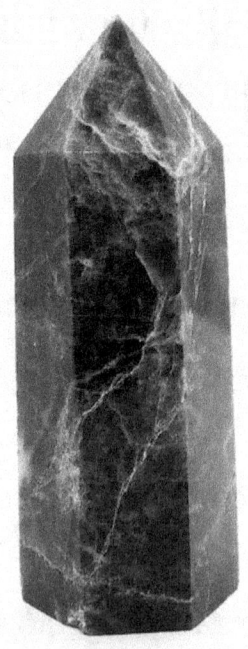

Sodalite is very easily obtained and can be found in Brazil, France, Greenland, Myanmar, North America, Romania, and Russia.

Appearance: this is a crystal that can be found in all sizes, and is mottled with light and dark blue. There can even be traces of blue-white. It is often sold as a tumbled stone.

Healing properties and uses: this crystal is beneficial towards the mind and can help improve your intuition and logical thinking. It connects to the third eye chakra and can be used for deep meditation. This stone encourages truth and idealism, improves the ability of a group to work together, and can remove confusion. It is a good stone to place near computers and other electrical devices as it has the ability to reduce electromagnetic pollution. It can encourage you to be more objective, rational and truthful, and helps your communication and the ability to express your emotions. Sodalite can be used to treat panic attacks, keep your mind calm and balance your emotions. It can further help you learn to trust and accept yourself and raises your self-esteem. It can be used to help balance your metabolism and strengthen your immune system, as well as lower fevers, help the body absorb liquids, and bring down blood pressure Sodalite is good for treating digestive and calcium disorders, insomnia, damage caused by radiation, and most problems regarding the throat.

Sunstone

This stone is found in Canada, Greece, India, Norway, and the United States. Although it isn't exceptionally rare or expensive, sunstone can only be found at stores specializing in this type of stone.

Appearance: this stone can either be transparent, or opaque with an iridescent surface. It tends to be a smaller crystal and is often sold as a tumbled stone.

Healing properties and uses: this crystal is full of positive energy and can bring feelings of joy and good nature towards others. It is strongly connected to the sun and its healing energy and light and can bring these elements into your meditation. It can also help clear all of your chakras. This stone can further help you get rid of unhealthy attachments to other people, especially if those people are very possessive. Sunstone can help you become more independent and say "no" to people from time to time. This stone can help you fight depression, increase your confidence by getting rid of hang-ups regarding occurrences such as being abandoned or discriminated against and break the bad habit of procrastinating. It can help you be more enthusiastic and optimistic and see things in a more positive way. It can be used together with the solar plexus chakra to remove repressed and emotions or emotions that weigh heavily on you. Sunstone encourages the body to heal itself and gives it the power to do so. It is beneficial to all the organs and nervous system and can be used to heal stomach ulcers and chronic sore throats. It is especially good at relieving general pains and aches throughout the body, rheumatism and cartilage problems. This stone was often associated with benevolent gods and spirits, and good luck.

Tiger's Eye

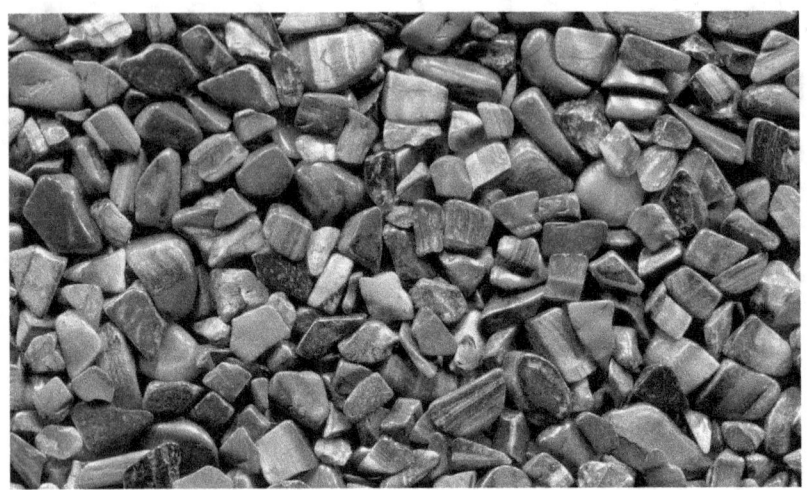

This stone is very easy to come by and is found in Australia, India, Mexico, South Africa, and the United States.

Appearance: this stone is striped and slightly shiny. It is usually a smaller type of stone that has a blue, brown-yellow, pink, or red color. It is most commonly sold as a tumbled stone.

Healing properties and uses: tiger's eye is strongly connected to both the earth and the sun. It is a grounding stone, but it also helps raise your spiritual energy. It can be used with the third eye chakra to develop and strengthen psychic abilities, or it can be used to balance the four lowest chakras in your body. This stone can help develop integrity and clarity, and it can help you find the power to achieve your goals. It can help you understand the difference between what you want and what you need, and can greatly help you become more committed in life. Tiger's eye is good for treating personality disorders and can help you gather scattered thoughts, improve your ability to see things in a practical way, and find quick solutions to most conflicts and dilemmas. It can help unblock the flow of energy, improve your self-confidence, and keep you from constantly criticizing yourself. It can also be used to lift your spirits and overcome depression, and can even balance the yin-yang energies within your body. Tiger's eye is used to treat broken bones and problems with the eyes, reproduction organs, throat, and constrictions. It also improves your night vision. In many cultures, the tradition exists to wear tiger's eye as a talisman that will protect the wearer from curses and ill-wishes.

Topaz

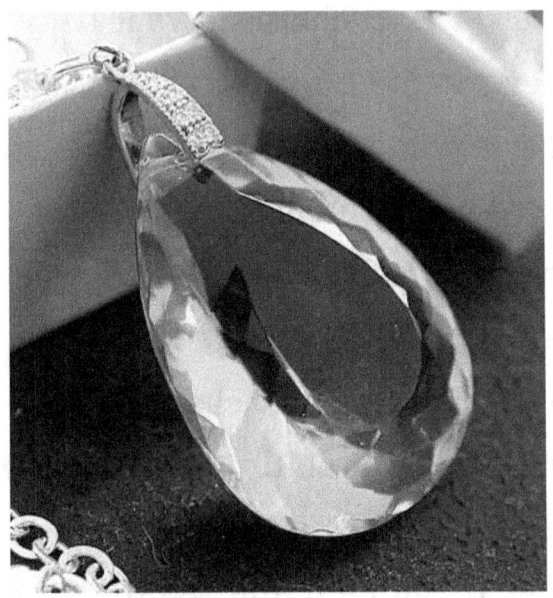

This is another stone that requires a specialized store, but aside from red-pink topaz, it isn't that rare. It is found in Australia, India, Mexico, Pakistan, South Africa, Sri Lanka, and the United States.

Appearance: topaz is a transparent crystal that grows into points. It can be either large or small, and the smaller crystals tend to be faceted. It can be blue, brown, colorless, golden-yellow, green or red-pink.

Healing properties and uses: this stone strongly connects to your sense of empathy and can direct its energy to whatever needs it the most. It can help you become more forgiving, trusting and truthful, and can get rid of feelings of uncertainty and doubt. Topaz can be used to cleanse your aura, encourage faster spiritual growth, and lessen tension. It is a very joyful and positive stone that can build your confidence and discover good personality traits and skills that are usually overlooked. It can remove all forms of negative energy and can help you better express your thoughts and ideas, making this a good stone for artists. It can make accepting love of any kind easier, and it provides emotional support when needed. Topaz is used to boost your general health, metabolism, and digestion. It can help steel your nerves, overcome anorexia, and improve your eyesight. It can also treat problems that affect your sense of taste.

Turquoise

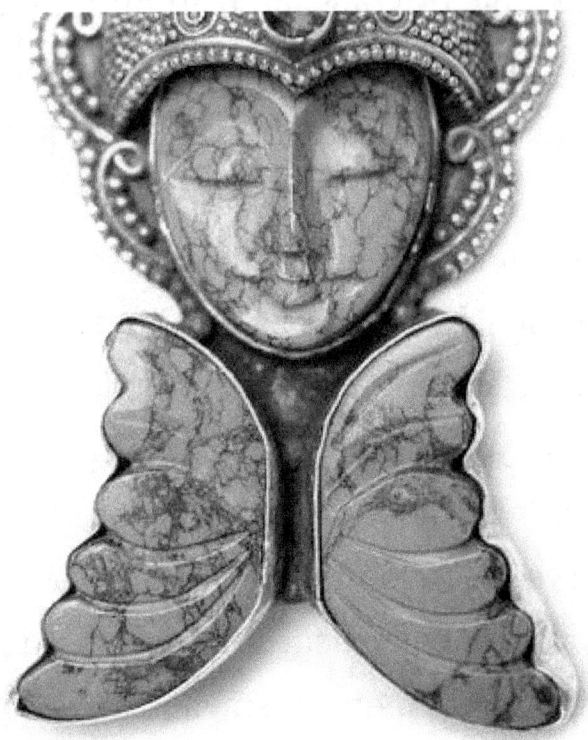

This stone isn't too hard to find and comes from Afghanistan, Arabia, China, Egypt, France, Iran, Mexico, Peru, Poland, Russia, Tibet, and the United States. It is a fairly valuable stone and is often faked.

Appearance: this stone is named after its color but can also be found in blue or green on occasion. It is an opaque stone that can be found in all sizes and often has dark veins. It is often sold as a polished stone.

Healing properties and uses: turquoise is excellent for healing both the body and soul. This stone is also fairly spiritual and can be used on the third eye chakra to strengthen your intuition and aid your meditation. It is good for removing both negative energy and pollutants in the air and can align all the chakras. Turquoise helps you find creative solutions to problems, removes nervousness in cases such as public speaking, and can help you develop balance and empathy. It is good for stabilizing intense mood swings, finding a strong inner calm, and expressing yourself in creatively. It can help treat depression, panic attacks and exhaustion, and can help strengthen feelings of romantic love. It is used to treat problems regarding the eyes, such as cataracts, stomach, gout, rheumatism and your immune system. It can remove acidity in the body, is good for bringing down inflammation, can lessen pain and cramps, remove toxins from the body and fight infections brought on by viruses. In ancient times, turquoise was believed to connect the power of the sea and sky with each other. It was worn as a protective amulet that changed color when danger was near.

Unakite

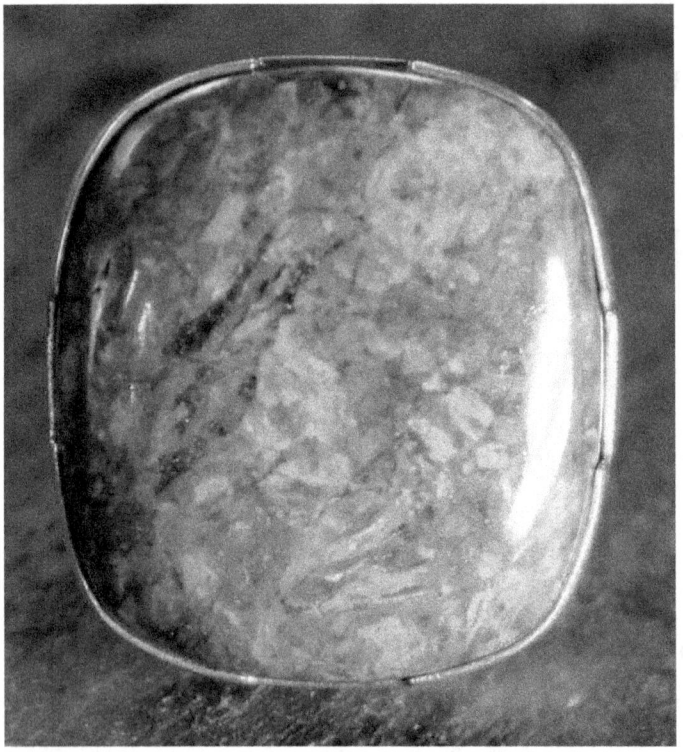

Unakite is very easy to come by and can be found in South Africa and the United States.

Appearance: this stone is mottled in dark green and yellowish-brown, with pinkish-red flecks. It is a fairly small type of stone and is most commonly sold as a tumbled stone.

Healing properties and uses: this is a grounding stone that works well with the third eye chakra and can be a good aide while meditating. It is also good for using together with other crystals. Unakite is good for placing in a room as either a single large piece or several smaller pieces to bring calmness and lessen electromagnetic pollution. It can help remove spiritual and psychological blockages that impede your growth in those areas. This crystal is often used to help rejuvenate those who have recently overcome any major illness and can be beneficial for the skin, hair, and reproductive system. It is often used to help ensure a healthy pregnancy and gain weight in cases where it is needed, such as anorexia or being underweight.

Variscite

This is stone is found in Austria, Bolivia, the Czech Republic, Germany, and the United States, and it can be bought from specialized stores.

Appearance: this is an opaque stone that can either be found as a large mass or on a matrix. It can be found in gray, green, and white, and can be veined at times.

Healing properties and uses: variscite can go a long way to provide encouragement, courage, and hope, and is often used to provide support for those who are ill or are considered invalids. This is a crystal that encourages unconditional love, clear thinking, and trust. It is very good for using together with the heart chakra, and can help overcome despair and sorrow. It can calm the nerves and help you become more comfortable with revealing your true self to the world around you. It can help bring out your more fun-loving and whimsical side, but can also partially protect you from the effects of alcohol for a time. Variscite can be used to keep your sleep peaceful and undisturbed by placing it under your pillow. It can help strengthen your perception and self-expression, and restores physical energy to your body. It is used to treat abdominal distension, gout, over acidity in the body, ulcers, gastritis, rheumatism, and problems with your nervous system. It can help restore and improve elasticity in the skin and veins, relieve cramps, and fight against male impotence.

Zoisite

This crystal can be acquired in specialized stores and is often found together with ruby. It is found in Austria, Cambodia, India, Kenya, Madagascar, Russia, Sri Lanka, and Tanzania.

Appearance: this is a very solid stone that is found in a single mass that can be practically any size. It has a reflective surface that can cause it to appear to have several colors and shades of the same color at once. Its colors are brown, blue, colorless, green, lavender-blue, pink, red, white and yellow.

Healing properties and uses: this crystal is good for transforming negative energy into positive energy.

It can help you stay in touch with who you are and can help you keep yourself from falling under peer pressure. It is good for helping deal with repressed emotions and can help dispel feelings of lethargy. It stimulates and encourage creativity and can help you regain your creative focus after an interruption. It can help support you during an illness or very stressful times, and it encourages the recovery process. Zoisite is used to remove toxins and unwanted acids from your body, reduce inflammation, improve your immune system, treat diseases and improves fertility. This stone acts slowly though is very beneficial towards the heart, lungs, pancreas, spleen, and cell regeneration. It is effective against diseases found in the ovaries and testicles and can be used together with ruby to strengthen potency.

References

A Brief History of Crystals and Healing. (n.d.). Retrieved from Crystal Age: https://www.crystalage.com/crystal_information/crystal_history/

Askinosie, H. (2014, November 5). *Chakra Healing with Crystals*. Retrieved from Energy Muse: https://www.energymuse.com/blog/chakra-healing-crystals/

Askinosie, H. (2015, November 20). *Meditation and Crystals for Kids*. Retrieved from Energy Muse: https://www.energymuse.com/blog/meditation-crystals-kids/

Color in Minerals. (n.d.). Retrieved from WebMineral: http://webmineral.com/help/Color.shtml#.XRQJoOgzZEZ

Coyle, C. (n.d.). *Animal WellnessGUide*. Retrieved from Crystal Healing for Animals: https://animalwellnessguide.com/crystal-healing-for-animals/

Crystal Lattice. (2019, June 9). Retrieved from Chemistry Libretext: https://chem.libretexts.org/Bookshelves/Physical_and_Theoretical_Chemistry_Textbook_Maps/Supplemental_Modules_(Physical_and_Theoretical_Chemistry)/Physical_Properties_of_Matter/States_of_Matter/Properties_of_Solids/Crystal_Lattice

Crystal Structure and Crystal System. (n.d.). Retrieved from Mineralogy: https://www.mpp.mpg.de/~bangert/Mineralogy/crystal.html

Crystal VAults. (n.d.). *Crystal Colors Explained*. Retrieved from Crystal Vaults: https://www.crystalvaults.com/crystal-colors-explained

Davis, F. (2018, June 21). *This is What Happens When Kids Use Crystals & Gemstones*. Retrieved from Cosmic Cuts: https://cosmiccuts.com/blogs/healing-stones-blog/crystals-and-gemstones-for-kids

Desy, P. I. (2019, May 2019). *How to Cleanse and Clear Your Crystals and Gemstones*. Retrieved from Learn Religions: https://www.learnreligions.com/cleanse-and-clear-your-crystals-1729392

Grundmann, M. (2008). *Crystal Balance*. Saarbreuken: Neue Erde GmbH.

Hall, J. (2003). *The Crystal Bible*. Hampshire: Godsfield Press Ltd.

Helmenstine, A. M. (2019, January 20). *What is a Crystal?* Retrieved from ThoughtCo.: https://www.thoughtco.com/what-is-a-crystal-607656

How do Crystals Form and Grow? (2016, March 11). Retrieved from Geology page: http://www.geologypage.com/2016/03/how-do-crystals-form-grow.html

HOW TO SPOT A FAKE CRYSTAL. (n.d.). Retrieved from KSKYE: http://www.kskyethelabel.com/how-to-spot-a-fake-crystal/

International Gem Society. (n.d.). *What is Gemstone Transparency?* Retrieved from International Gem Society: https://www.gemsociety.org/article/gemstone-transparency/

Lazzerini, E. (2018, September 11). *Crystal Shapes & What They mean.* Retrieved from Ethan Lazzerini - Crystal Blog, Guides & Tips: https://www.ethanlazzerini.com/crystal-shapes-meanings/

Mildon, E. (n.d.). *The Crystal Grid Is The Key To Unlocking Your Inner Badass.* Retrieved from mbgmindfulness:

https://www.mindbodygreen.com/articles/crystal-grid-how-to

Mindvalley. (2017, December 20). *The Complete Guide to the 7 Chakras - For BEginners*. Retrieved from Mindvalley: https://blog.mindvalley.com/7-chakras/

Mineral Properties: Color. (n.d.). Retrieved from Minerals.net: https://www.minerals.net/resource/property/color.aspx

Rekstis, E. (2018, June 21). *Healing Crystals 101*. Retrieved from healthline: https://www.healthline.com/health/mental-health/guide-to-healing-crystals#1

Shannon. (2018, October 5). *Crystal Shapes: What they Mean and How to Use them*. Retrieved from Spirit Earth Magazine: https://www.spiritearthmag.org/2018/10/05/crystal-shapes-what-they-mean/

Shine, T. (2018, September 10). *A Beginner's Guide to Clearing, Cleansing and Charging Crystals.* Retrieved from healthline: https://www.healthline.com/health/how-to-cleanse-crystals

www.ingramcontent.com/pod-product-compliance
Lightning Source LLC
Chambersburg PA
CBHW062143280526
45788CB00001B/290